HERE'S HOW THIS BOOK HAS HELPED OTHERS...

"All of us who have been diagnosed with Parkinson's owe you great gratitude for all the work and effort you have put into compiling all the information you have to date. It is truly astounding.

You know well the shock of being told one has, what at least for the present, is an incurable and slow growing illness. Thank God for you as it is a great encouragement to know first that one is not alone and secondly that you have dedicated so much, initially for your mother and now for all of us.

May God continue to bless and reward you."

- Frank

"I have gotten more from your book than anything else about Parkinson's. It is a terrible disease but people like you and your knowledge are making it liveable. Thank You."

- Suzanne

"I want you to know your book is wonderful. I have learned a lot from it and it is very informative. I've enjoyed reading your book so much. Now I don't feel so alone knowing I'm not the only one who has Parkinson's. I feel your book will help my family to understand more about how I feel and understand what Parkinson's is. Thanks for your book."

- Monica

"Thank you so very much. Your book was a huge help and a wealth of information, which stayed my worries and fears. Thank you from my heart."

- Allen

"Thank you again for making such a wonderful tribute to your mom (and thank her for the "inside track"!!). She must be utterly thrilled that you are bringing such knowledge and good information to PD/parkinsonism sufferers around the world. Well done you!"

- Joanne

"Your work has helped me so very much in the progress of this challenging and sometimes overwhelming trial. Your willingness to share your life's stories, do the research in so many of the difficult areas, and put forth the dire effort to communicate all of that to a tremendously diverse population is quite commendable.

You have changed, and by that I mean dramatically helped, my life personally and for that no amount of thanks is adequate. You have equipped so many to find the courage to press on. Thank you for you, as well as for your sharing heart."

- Rusty

"I really appreciate you making this book available. I have made a good effort to be knowledgeable about Parkinson's and it is difficult to find it all in one place. You have done that. I believe in being well informed and believe that knowledge is power. Thank you for sharing with the world your findings and caring enough about your Mom to do the research that you have done. God Bless you abundantly."

- Justine

"Thanks Lianna. I have read part of your book and passed it onto my Mum as it is my Dad who has just been diagnosed. We are so grateful that you have made your story available and have such helpful and understanding answers to many questions that are not always answered by the medical profession in the right way. Keep up your outstanding work. Warmest Thanks."

- Rick and Family

"With your good work in organizing the results of your research and discovery, you have provided a worthwhile service that will benefit countless individuals. Your efforts are very much appreciated. Thank you."

-Peter

"Your book has such warmth and optimism, exactly what I needed at this point. Enough with the medical journals. You give us just the info we need. The whole family appreciates it! When I lost it your website for PD/caregivers, my heart dropped. Good thing you created such a catchy address.

Blessings to you and your mother."

- Elaine

"Just a few lines to let you know how much I have appreciated your book, it has given me a far greater insight into the disease. After reading it I now realize I must have been carrying the symptoms around without knowing it. Your book has highlighted all these symptoms and to me has taken all the mystery out of it and makes me feel better and more able to cope with it.

I would like you to know that I am truly grateful for the effort and time you put in to your book and once again thank you, I have thoroughly enjoyed it and hope to hear from you again soon. Please give my regards to your mom, all the way from New Zealand."

- John

"Many thanks. We are working our way through your book, which is proving to be so very helpful in answering questions left unanswered from the professionals. My brother-in-law has recently been diagnosed with Parkinson's disease but already he is some way down the road of the disease, mobile but only just. With the help of your own experience we are hoping to look forward with a far more positive attitude than that we had when it was first diagnosed.

Thank you so very much."

- Julie

"I have received your book, and read it cover to cover as well as the other bonuses. You have a well written and useful book for those of us who struggle with this disease day in and day out.

I can tell you that I have a medical background as a trauma nurse, and that I had no idea what and how this disease was going to affect me. Your book provided me some new avenues to pursue. I appreciate the input and your time."

- Laura

"Thank you for your book. I have now started to read it and am really pleased with the information you provide. It is so easy to understand and a very great help and reassurance. I hope your mom is managing to cope. She is fortunate to have a daughter like you.

Thank you Lianna and God bless you."

- Heather

EVERYTHING
YOU NEED TO KNOW
ABOUT
PARKINSON'S
DISEASE

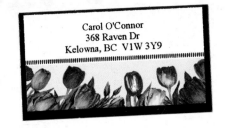

EVERYTHING YOU NEED TO KNOW ABOUT PARKINSON'S DISEASE

THE
TOP 100
QUESTIONS
ABOUT
PARKINSON'S
DISEASE

Lianna Marie

Printed by CafePress.com in the United States of America.

Visit our website at www.allaboutparkinsons.com

It is not the purpose of this publication to reprint all the information that is otherwise available about Parkinson's Disease, but to compliment, amplify, and supplement other sources of information. You should NOT rely solely upon the information, content or opinions within this publication.

Rather, you are urged to read all the available material, learn as much as possible about Parkinson's Disease and tailor the information to your individual needs.

Every effort has been made to make the information contained herein as accurate as possible. Also note that although this publication is updated often, medical information changes rapidly. Therefore, please be advised some information may be out of date and there may be errors, both typographical and in content. Therefore, this publication should only be used as a general guide and not as the ultimate source of Parkinson's Disease information.

In no way should this publication be considered as offering medical advice! The content in this publication is presented in summary form, is general in nature, and is provided for informational purposes only.

The information in this publication is provided for educational and informational purposes only, and is not intended to be a substitute for a health care provider's consultation. Please consult your own physician or appropriate health care provider about the applicability of any opinions or recommendations with respect to your own symptoms or medical conditions as these diseases commonly present with variable signs and symptoms.

The information in this publication should not be considered complete, nor should it be relied on to suggest a course of treatment for a particular individual. It should not be used in place of a visit, call, consultation or the advice of your physician or other qualified health care provider.

Always consult with your physician or other qualified health care provider before embarking on a new treatment, diet or fitness program. You should never disregard medical advice or delay in seeking it because of something you have read in this publication.

The Author, Publisher, and any contributing parties specifically disclaim any liability, loss, or risk that is incurred as a consequence, directly or indirectly, of the use and application of any contents of this work.

First Edition Published 2006.

ISBN 0-978-20130-2

To my mom,

my number one fan.

Thank you for

encouraging me

caring for me

loving me...

Now it's my turn.

ACKNOWLEDGEMENTS

First, to God, for without Him, none of this would have been possible.

To mom, again, thanks for sharing your stories and tips so that others may be able to live healthier and happier lives.

To Dave, thanks for caring for mom and sharing your ideas and advice with other caregivers.

And last but not least, to Mark, thanks for all your hard work and all-nighters that went into helping me put this book together. Your love and encouragement are so much appreciated. I can't thank you enough.

CONTENTS

Some Words You Need to Know

Antioxidant: a chemical that prevents damage to cells in your body

Bradykinesia: slowness of movement

Dopamine: a chemical substance (neurotransmitter) found in the brain that sends impulses from one nerve cell to another and regulates movement, balance, and walking; the substance that is lost in PD

Dopamine Agonist: drugs that imitate the effects of dopamine

Dyskinesia: the most common and disruptive side-effect of PD medications; an involuntary movement that can accompany peak doses of levodopa

Levodopa: the most effective anti-Parkinson drug which is changed into dopamine in the brain and usually combined with carbidopa as Sinemet

Neurologist: a specialist in the diagnosis and treatment of disorders of the nervous system (*In this book we often use the word doctor instead of neurologist)

Off Time: when people with Parkinson's have a decrease in their ability to move and have other symptoms that make it hard to get up from a chair, to speak, walk, or perform their usual activities (*can also be called "down" time); happens because the person's dose of levodopa has worn off too soon or has suddenly and unexpectedly stopped working.

Parkinsonian or Parkie: a person with Parkinson's disease

PD: short form for Parkinson's disease

PARKINSON' S EXPLAINED

What is Parkinson's?

To put it simply, Parkinson's is a disease that affects the functioning of a small part of the brain.

Basically what happens is that certain nerve cells in that small part of the brain (the part called the "substantia nigra") start to degenerate and when they do a chemical in the brain called dopamine is lost.

Dopamine is a chemical that helps transmit signals or messages from the brain to different parts of the body. Because the dopamine is reduced and the brain can't send the signals as well, this causes problems with body movement in someone with Parkinson's.

Unfortunately, the sad part about Parkinson's disease is that it is a disease that is long lasting and gets worse over time.

However, the good news is that because the disease usually progresses slowly, it often takes years before there is a serious impact on a person's quality of life.

What is the History of Parkinson's?

Parkinson's disease is named after an English doctor and writer named James Parkinson who first described the disease.

He wrote a paper about the disease which was published in 1817. This was the first time in history that someone described the symptoms of this disease in depth.

His paper was called "Essay on the Shaking Palsy" and to this day Parkinson's disease is still sometimes called the "shaking palsy".

What Causes It?

In short, we don't know yet. There are many theories about the possible causes of Parkinson's, but none of them have been proven yet. Most people researching the disease agree that there are probably multiple factors that contribute to someone getting Parkinson's.

A lot of people ask about things like heredity, pesticides, head trauma (as in Muhammed Ali's case), and aging, and whether or not these could be possible causes for Parkinson's.

First of all, let's start with what the researchers do know. They do know that Parkinson's does not result from something that a person has done, from his or her diet, or from stress.

Head trauma is also something that researchers know rarely causes Parkinson's. Some studies have found though, that those who have experienced a head injury are four times more likely to develop PD than those who have never suffered a head injury.

The same studies showed that the risk of PD increases by 8 times for people who required hospitalization for head trauma and 11 times for those people who had a loss of consciousness, skull fracture, prolonged memory loss or more complications. Even though the association is strong, researchers warn that this doesn't mean that head injuries cause PD. The same is true for tumours.

Researchers also know that heredity does not play a major role in causing the disease except in familial Parkinson's disease (families with many members having the disease over several generations). Basically, if you have a family member who has Parkinson's, it is most likely a coincidence if you happen to develop the disease as well (because the disease is so common).

Researchers have discovered that it is possible that some people have a genetic susceptibility to developing Parkinson's disease. What that means is that for example, some people just don't have the ability to deal with toxic materials, so when they are exposed to them, they may develop PD.

Speaking of toxic materials, this is an area in which researchers searching for possible causes of Parkinson's are currently very interested in.

Researchers have suggested that Parkinson's might result from a toxin that gradually builds up in the brain, causing the degeneration of certain nerve cells in that small part of the brain we talked about earlier called the substantia nigra.

This toxin could build up either through exposure to an environmental toxin or as a by-product of a process of the brain. It could also be possible that people get the disease from exposure to a toxin early in life, combined with factors related to aging.

Unfortunately, there still is no firm evidence that environmental toxic materials such as industrial pollutants, herbicides, and pesticides may cause Parkinson's. Researchers will have to continue to work on this one....

Finally, in regards to aging, there is evidence that the number of nerve cells in the substantia nigra decreases as a natural part of aging. Maybe Parkinson's is related to aging then? But what about all those people who are in their 50's, 40's or younger with Parkinson's?

Researchers have considered that maybe there is some kind of accelerated aging process taking place in the brains of people with Parkinson's, but what the process is or how it starts is still unclear.

Who Gets It?

Here are some quick facts about who Parkinson's affects:

- it is estimated that 6.3 million people have the disease world wide

- about 1 to 1.5 million Americans have the disease

- 1 in 1000 people develop the disease

- 1 in 100 people over the age of 65 develop the disease

- 1 in 50 people over the age of 80 develop the disease

- 60 is the average age of developing the disease

- about 1 in 7 people with Parkinson's develop it before the age of 40 ("Early-Onset Parkinson's Disease")

- in Early-Onset Parkinson's, the disease develops between the ages of 21 and 40

- men and women are equally likely to develop Parkinson's (although some studies say men may be slightly more likely)

- all ethnic groups and occupations are about equally affected by PD

How Do I Know if I Have Parkinson's?

In order to really know if you have Parkinson's you need to be diagnosed. The process of diagnosis usually begins with you contacting your family doctor who will usually refer you to a neurologist or geriatrician.

The neurologist will take the history of the development of the symptoms from you and conduct a neurological exam. You might also be recommended to take some lab tests that will help determine if you have a different condition that may be similar to Parkinson's, but really is not. For example, there are tremors that are not related to Parkinson's.

There is still no one specific test that helps in the diagnosis of Parkinson's. Diagnosis comes from being examined by your neurologist and by ruling out other possible causes for your symptoms.

What made my mom decide to go to the doctor originally was the tremor she was experiencing in her right hand. Obviously, she knew this was not "normal" so she went to get it checked out.

Unfortunately at the time (over 17 years ago), the doctor dismissed it because he said she was too young to have Parkinson's (she was 48). Nowadays though, Early-Onset Parkinson's is well known to doctors so she probably would have been diagnosed much sooner (it took 3 years for her to finally be diagnosed).

Though she did not realize it at the time, there were other additional symptoms that she was experiencing before her diagnosis that were the first signs of Parkinson's. She did not know that these were linked to her having the disease until after she started learning about the signs and symptoms, after her diagnosis.

Other than her obvious hand tremor, she said she knew there was something different in her walk. She noticed that her feet seemed to hit the floor differently and that there was more wear and tear on the heel of her right shoe.

She also noticed dryness in her eyes which she later found out was due to the fact that people with Parkinson's don't blink as often. Another thing that happened was that her sense of smell was not as good as it normally was.

My mom always had a keen sense of smell so this was more obvious to her. She later read an article in Reader's Digest that said that the loss of sense of smell is one of the first signs that appears in people with Parkinson's.

Finally, the last things she noticed were while she was at work. One was the fact that her handwriting was not round and fluid anymore, but rather "tight" or tense looking. The other thing she noticed at work was as she calls it, her "scatter brain". She would often find herself starting a project then putting it down and moving on to another before it was finished.

These symptoms experienced by my mom are all common to someone who is being diagnosed with Parkinson's, but there are others as well (check out the answer to **Question #28: "What are the most common symptoms?" p. 25**). Remember that every person is different and so are the number and types of signs and symptoms that one would expect to see before diagnosis.

What convinced my mom's neurologist that she had the disease was when he asked her to walk and he noticed that her one arm didn't swing like the other (it actually stopped swinging). This is also a sign that many people with Parkinson's have.

It is important to keep in mind that there are several **Parkinson's "look-alikes" (see Question #16: "Are there different types of Parkinson's?" p. 13**) and in the end, it is the neurologist who will ultimately need to tell you or your loved one if you have Parkinson's disease.

Is it Hereditary?

As mentioned earlier, researchers say that heredity does not play a major role in causing the disease except in familial Parkinson's disease (families with many members having the disease over several generations).

Even with familial Parkinson's disease though, studies show that in most of the cases, the inheritance factor is not of major importance.

It's been found that about 5 to 7 percent of people with Parkinson's have a relative with the disease. This percentage is no higher than we'd expect from chance alone. Basically, if you have a sister, brother, mother, father, uncle, or aunt, etc., who has Parkinson's it would only be a coincidence if you also got the disease.

A recent study of twins showed that Parkinson's disease before age 50 is strongly genetic. The same study did not find genetics to be a factor in Parkinson's disease after age 50, but this finding is not a hundred percent certain.

Where Does it Start?

Parkinson's disease starts in the small part of the brain called the substantia nigra. The symptoms of the disease develop when the levels of the chemical messenger dopamine are reduced by about 80 percent.

How Fast Does it Progress?

This is a hard question to answer. It really varies from one person to another. The time between when the symptoms first appear to severe disability can vary between 3 and 30 or more years.

Sometimes the disease will remain static (doesn't change) for the first ten years (happens in about 5 to 10 percent of cases) and sometimes severe disability can occur within a few years (happens in about 6 to15 percent of cases). Most people with the disease will have a progression that falls somewhere in between these two extremes.

Some studies have shown that people with Parkinson's whose first symptom was a tremor and whose main symptom has remained a tremor have experienced a slow progression in the disease (this probably accounts for about 5 to 10 percent of all cases).

I know this was a question my mom asked her neurologist almost immediately after diagnosis. It took a while for him to give her what she calls a "straight answer" but when he finally did he said that she could expect to have a major disability within 10 years.

She was diagnosed at 51 and had to take a disability pension from her work at the age of 62 so I guess the doc was pretty accurate in my mom's case.

Is There Any Way to Slow the Progression of the Disease?

First of all, the diagnosis part of Parkinson's is very important. New research says that if you can catch the disease very early on, often something can be done to delay the progression.

The sooner you can start treating the disease with proper medication, the better. Starting on the drug Deprenyl (selegiline) early in the disease can possibly slow the progression down.

There is some controversy about the use of Deprenyl though. Although it is possible that Deprenyl may help slow the progression of the disease early on, not all researchers agree.

I know Mom sometimes feels a bit sad about the fact that it took so long (3 years) for her to get diagnosed and started on treatment. She wonders how much she might have delayed the progression of her PD had she known she had the disease sooner.

There have been many studies on various new drugs, nutrients, vitamins, etc., which have all been trying to figure out if this disease can be slowed down.

There was a study at Emory University and nine other centres nationwide a couple of years ago. In it, researchers found that the naturally occurring compound coenzyme Q10 could slow the progression of PD in its early stages by up to 44 percent. Research is still ongoing into this.

Vitamins C, E, and selenium have also been linked to possibly helping slow the progression of the disease.

Finally, more recent studies have shown that a new drug called Rasagiline may also slow the progression of Parkinson's disease, but it is still too early to tell.

Mom's doctor has always encouraged her to try vitamins and herbs to see if they help. He says they can't hurt, so why not? Why not ask your doctor if you think some of these things might help you?

You might also want to check out **Question #73: "What alternative treatments are available for PD?" (p. 65)** to see if there might be any other alternative treatments you may want to talk to your doctor about.

Are Some Cases Worse Than Others?

Yes! Everybody's different, but in general people with Parkinson's who have a tremor tend to have a milder type of Parkinson's.

Some people (especially those who have a tremor in one arm) may have a very mild form of the disease and require no treatment for several years.

Mom had a tremor in one hand for at least three years without any other major symptoms. Also, her doctor has been very surprised at how slow the progression has been to the left side of her body. She has only recently noticed slight tremors in her left hand and this is over 17 years after her diagnosis.

What Are the Stages of Parkinson's?

Two doctors named Dr. Hoehn and Dr. Yahr developed a scale that puts Parkinson's disease into five stages. The first stage is the mildest stage of the disease and stage five is the worst stage.

The symptoms may be mild or severe or happen a lot, or not as much. Also, the time spent at each stage of the disease varies, and the skipping of stages, from Stage 1 to Stage 3, for example, is not uncommon.

Stage 1 The main symptoms- tremor, muscle stiffness, slowness of movement and problems with posture- are only on one side of the body. Problems with balance might also appear.

Stage 2 The disease will be on both sides of the body now and minor symptoms like problems with swallowing, talking and something called "facial masking" (loss of facial expression) may be noticed.

Stage 3 The same symptoms of Stage 2 are still there but may be worse now. Problems with balance will now be noticed for the first time. At this stage, the person with PD is still independent.

Stage 4 The person with PD will now be getting more and more disabled and will need help with some or all activities of daily living.

Stage 5 At this stage the person is confined to a wheelchair or bed and needs total assistance.

Do People Die from Parkinson's?

No, people do not die from Parkinson's. People with the disease die of the same causes as do other people of the same age.

You may have heard someone say "so and so died of Parkinson's...", but this is not true. They may have died of complications related to the disease, but the disease itself is not the official cause of death.

One interesting fact is that people with Parkinson's are less likely to die of cancer, maybe because they are less likely to smoke.

What is the Life Expectancy of Someone With PD?

With proper treatment, the life expectancy of people with Parkinson's is about the same as the general population (currently about 77 years but varies depending on what country you live in).

Some studies suggest that life expectancy is somewhat affected, but more recent estimates say that it remains within six months of normal life expectancy. (That's good news!)

Can Parkinson's Be Prevented?

To date, there is no known prevention or cure for Parkinson's disease. There are, however, several treatment options, including drug therapy and/or surgery that can reduce the symptoms, and make living with the disease easier.

How Long Can a Person With Parkinson's Expect to Keep Their Independence?

Again, everyone is different, and the best person to ask this question to is your neurologist. Most people (including my mom who was diagnosed at 51) live many years after diagnosis without experiencing any major disabilities.

It's a good idea to talk to your doctor/neurologist regularly in an open and honest way about your symptoms and how you are feeling. This will help him or her to help you best achieve the maximum out of your medications and hopefully extend the length of time in which you can remain independent.

When my mom was first diagnosed, a family member suggested she go to a meeting for people with Parkinson's. When she got there, she encountered a room full of people in wheel chairs. This was very discouraging for her (and probably not the best idea for a newly-diagnosed person to do!).

She decided at that moment that she was going to do all that she could to keep her independence for as long as possible. She explained to me that though today she often likes the choice of say using a scooter to get around a shopping mall, she doesn't want to feel that she has to be in that scooter.

"Don't let anyone take away your independence", my mom says. In other words, don't give up and say, "Oh well, I have Parkinson's. I guess I'm doomed to being in that wheelchair."

Her advice is to keep doing as much as you can for as long as you can without causing you and yours too much stress. Obviously, if something can be done in a few minutes that is taking you an hour, don't be so stubborn as to not ask for help.

Are There Different Types of Parkinson's?

#1   Yes, there are two main types of Parkinson's disease. The main type, idiopathic or primary Parkinson's disease is what about 76 percent of all people with PD have. In this type, the cause of the disease is unknown.

People with this type of Parkinson's are diagnosed when they have 3 of the 5 main symptoms (resting tremor, rigidity, bradykinesia, problems with posture, and walking problems) and there is no history of injury or illness or any other known cause of the symptoms, and when there is a good response to levodopa therapy.

#2   The second type, called secondary Parkinsonism, is what the remaining 24 percent of people with PD have. In this type, there are other causes for the disease and they are therefore considered to have Parkinsonism secondary to another illness or known cause.

Here are the two types of Parkinson's and some descriptions of the different forms of Secondary Parkinsonism:

1. IDIOPATHIC OR PRIMARY PARKINSON'S DISEASE

2. SECONDARY PARKINSONISM:

- **Postencephalitic Parkinsonism**

Back around the time of World War 1, there was a viral disease called encephalitis lethargica that attacked almost 5 million people throughout the world, and then suddenly disappeared in the 1920s.

The disease was known as sleeping sickness in the United States and it killed one third of the people who got it and in many others it led to post-encephalitic Parkinsonism.

This postencephalitic Parkinsonism was a pretty severe form of movement disorder in which some patients developed disabling neurological disorders.

(In 1973, neurologist Oliver Sacks published "Awakenings", which was an account of his work in the late 1960's with surviving post-encephalitic patients in a New York hospital. Using the then-experimental drug levodopa, Dr. Sacks was able to temporarily "awaken" these patients from their statue-like state. There's also a movie by the same name that was released in 1990)

- **Drug-induced Parkinsonism**

This form of Parkinson's is reversible and sometimes results from use of certain drugs (ex. chlorpromazine and haloperidol) that are used for psychiatric patients.

Some drugs used for stomach disorders (metoclopramide) and high blood pressure (reserpine) may also produce parkinsonian symptoms. Stopping the medication or lowering the dosage causes the symptoms to go away.

- **Striatonigral Degeneration**

In this form of Parkinsonism, the substantia nigra is only mildly affected, while other brain areas show more severe damage than occurs in patients with primary Parkinson's disease.

People with this type of Parkinsonism tend to show more rigidity and the disease progresses more rapidly.

- **Arteriosclerotic Parkinsonism/Vascular Parkinsonism**

This type of Parkinson's is sometimes known as pseudoparkinsonism. It involves damage to brain vessels due to multiple small strokes.

You probably won't see tremor in this type of Parkinsonism, but you most likely will see dementia (loss of mental skills and abilities).

Drugs used to treat Parkinson's don't really help people with this type of Parkinson's.

- **Toxin-induced Parkinsonism**

Some toxins like manganese dust, carbon disulfide, and carbon monoxide can also cause Parkinsonism. A chemical known as MPTP (methyl-phenyl-tetrahydropyridine) causes a permanent form of Parkinsonism that closely resembles Parkinson's disease.

Researchers discovered this reaction in the 1980s when heroin addicts in California who had taken an illicit street drug contaminated with MPTP started to develop severe Parkinsonism.

MPTP-induced Parkinsonism is very rapid in its onset (as quick as a few days to full symptoms), whereas idiopathic PD has a slow progression and may take years to become evident.

- **Parkinsonism-Dementia Complex of Guam**

This form occurs among the Chamorro populations of Guam and the Mariana Islands and may be accompanied by a disease resembling amyotrophic lateral sclerosis (Lou Gehrig's disease).

The progression of this disease is fast, with people usually dying within 5 years. Some researchers wonder if there might be an environmental cause, like the use of flour from the highly toxic seed of the cycad plant.

This flour was a dietary staple for many years when rice and other food supplies were unavailable in this region, especially during World War II. Other studies, however, disagree with this link.

- **Parkinsonism Accompanying Other Conditions**

Parkinsonian symptoms may also appear in patients with other, neurological disorders such as Shy-Drager syndrome (sometimes called multiple system atrophy), progressive supranuclear palsy, Wilson's disease, Huntington's disease, Hallervorden-Spatz syndrome, Alzheimer's disease, diffuse Lewy body disease, Creutzfeldt-Jakob disease, olivopontocerebellar atrophy, and post-traumatic encephalopathy.

- **Parkinsonism Due to Other Causes**

Parkinsonism symptoms may also appear as a result of boxing, other head trauma, and hydrocephalus (an abnormal accumulation of cerebrospinal fluid (CSF) within cavities called ventricles inside the brain).

What is Idiopathic Parkinson's?

Idiopathic Parkinson's disease is the most common form of Parkinson's, also called primary or classic Parkinson's.

Parkinson's disease is called idiopathic Parkinson's because the cause is unknown. In the other forms of Parkinson's, a cause is known or suspected.

What is Parkinson's Plus?

Parkinson's Plus disorders are like cousins of Parkinson's disease. They're called Parkinson's Plus because they are disorders that have similar symptoms to Parkinson's.

Many people get these Parkinson Plus disorders and think they have Parkinson's but actually do not. These disorders are different from idiopathic PD.

Some examples of Parkinson Plus disorders are:

- Multiple-system atrophy (MSA)

- Progressive supranuclear palsy (PSP)

- Shy-Drager syndrome

- Striatonigral degeneration

- Parkinsonism-dementia-ALS complex

- Corticobasat degeneration

- Autosomal dominant Lewy body disease

- Alzheimer's disease

- Wilson's disease

- Guam disease

Some of the major ways in which Parkinson's Plus is different from idiopathic Parkinson's are as follows:

1. Levodopa therapy rarely works with PD Plus syndromes

2. PD Plus syndromes show additional symptoms that people with PD don't have. For example, in Corticobasat degeneration, there is the alien limb phenomenon (not feeling in control of the activities of an arm or leg)

3. There isn't a resting tremor in PD Plus and people often experience falls early on in the disorder

What is Lewy Body Disease?

Lewy body disease is a kind of dementia. Dementia is a general decline in cognitive abilities (thinking, memory, language, etc.).

There are many kinds of dementia. The most common and best known kind is Alzheimer's disease. Lewy body disease is thought to be the second most common kind of dementia. It causes cognitive problems similar to those seen in Alzheimer's disease and motor problems like those in Parkinson's.

Lewy body disease is currently incurable and it gets worse with time.

Lewy body disease is also referred to as dementia with Lewy bodies, Lewy body dementia, diffuse Lewy body disease, senile dementia of Lewy body type, and Lewy body variant of Alzheimer's disease.

The following are some of the symptoms of Lewy Body Disease:

- cognitive problems (problems with thinking, memory, language, etc.)

- motor problems like Parkinson's disease (but not as severe), difficulties in walking are the most common problem

- muscle stiffness and a tendency to fall are common

- tremor less common

- periods of being alert and coherent alternate with periods of being confused and unresponsive to questions

- visual hallucinations (usually occurring early on) and delusions

What is Essential Tremor and How is it Different from PD?

Essential tremor (ET) is the most common cause of tremor (involuntary shaking). It is a condition that affects the muscles of the hands, arms, head and sometimes the voice.

Essential tremor does not affect life expectancy, but things like writing and eating can become very difficult.

ET does not increase the risk for Parkinson's disease but the condition is often mistaken for Parkinson's. Although ET is 10-20 times more common than PD, people with essential tremor can go on to develop Parkinson's disease (but how many do so isn't known).

Both essential tremor (ET) and Parkinson's disease (PD) are movement disorders and are sometimes associated because they have similar features. A movement disorder can be defined as any disease or injury that interferes with an individual's movement.

Symptoms of Essential Tremor vs. Symptoms of Parkinson's (highlighted):

- tremors that get worse with purposeful movement (action tremor) / **have resting tremor (tremor gets worse at rest)**

- nodding head (head tremor) / **tremor may involve the chin, but rarely the head**

- fast tremor (4 to 12Hz)/ **tremor not as fast**

- tremor is usually bilateral (on both sides of the body) / **tremor starts on one side only then eventually progresses to the other side**

- tremors are the only symptom/ **tremors are only one of many symptoms of PD**

- difficulty with balance is rare/ **loss of balance and increased falls is common in people with Parkinson's**

- tremor can usually be relieved temporarily with ingestion of small amounts of alcohol/ **tremor is not usually relieved by alcohol**

- tremor does not respond to antiparkinsonian medication/ **tremor does respond to antiparkinsonian medication**

- a pill-rolling quality is usually not present in tremor/ **pill rolling quality is present**

- doesn't cause other health problems/ **is associated with a stooped posture, reduced rigid limbs, slow movement, a shuffling gait, speech problems other than tremor and sometimes memory loss**

- minor loss of sense of smell/ **loss of sense of smell is more significant**

- family history of ET usually exists/ **family history of PD doesn't usually exist**

What Percentage of People With PD Do Not Have a Tremor?

If PD starts without signs of tremor, it is likely to be more severe than if tremor had been present. Up to 25 percent of people with Parkinson's disease do not have tremor.

Does Age Play a Role in Getting Parkinson's?

Age is one of the main risk factors for Parkinson's disease. Although the disease can affect adults in their 20's, it usually starts in middle or late life. The risk continues to increase with age.

Some researchers think that people with Parkinson's disease may have damage within their brains from genetic or environmental factors that becomes worse over time.

Are There Look-Alike Conditions that Have Similar Symptoms to Parkinson's?

Yes, there are several "Look-Alikes" to Parkinson's. A number of people first diagnosed with Parkinson's may have these instead.

Here are some of the conditions that can sometimes be confused for Parkinson's:

- **Benign Essential Tremor:**

This is a common condition that may appear in older people and slowly progress over the years. The tremor is usually equal in both hands and increases when the patient stretches their hands out in front of them or when their hands are moving.

The tremor may involve the head but not the legs. People with Benign Tremor have no other Parkinson's symptoms, and there is usually a family history of tremor.

Parkinsonian Tremor and Benign Tremor generally respond to different drugs. A small number of people with Benign Essential Tremor (less than five percent) develop PD.

- **Shy Drager Syndrome (Multiple System Atrophy):**

This is a condition in which the earliest and most severe symptoms are dizziness on standing, bladder difficulty, and impotence.

These autonomic symptoms are followed by PD symptoms such as rigidity, tremor, bradykinesia, problems with posture, and gait difficulty.

- **Normal Pressure Hydrocephalus:**

This is a pretty uncommon condition where the person has difficulty walking, has mental changes (like forgetfulness), and bladder problems.

The condition is caused by an enlargement of the fluid cavities (called ventricles) in the brain which compress the parts of the brain that help you think and walk.

There is no known cause of Normal Pressure Hydrocephalus. The condition may be helped by a shunt (a tube placed in the ventricle which drains off the excessive fluid and carries it away).

- **Striato-Nigral Degenereation:**

This is also an uncommon disorder in which people become stiff and slow and develop difficulties with balance and walking.

Usually people do not have tremor and it's hard to tell if they have this condition or PD just by giving them a neurological exam. One thing that will be different between the two conditions is that people with Striato-Nigral Degenaration will not respond to Levadopa.

Only after the person dies can you tell if the person had this disorder or PD because in Striato-Nigral Degeneration most of the damage is in the Striatum part of the brain and not the Substantia Nigra (like in PD).

- **Pseudobulbar Palsy:**

This is a common disorder that happens in people with disease of the blood vessels of the brain (Arteriosclerosis). Arteriosclerosis is especially likely to happen in people with high blood pressure or diabetes.

People develop Pseudobulbar Palsy as a result of having many small strokes (ministrokes), most of which are so mild that they are unaware of them.

The ministrokes usually damage the part of the brain that controls balance and walking, the same area involved in PD.

You may not be able to tell the difference between these two disorders by a neurological exam alone, but people with Pseudobulbar Palsy do not respond to antiparkinsonian drugs.

- **Progressive Supernuclear Palsy:**

This is an uncommon disorder where people develop paralysis of their eye movements, difficulty in speaking, rigidity, and senility.

People with this disorder experience changes in the brain that are similar to those of PD, but are greater. Antiparkinson drugs don't work as treatment for this disorder.

- **Wilson's Disease:**

This is a rare inherited disorder that happens to people below the age of 40, and involves damage to the brain and the liver. Early diagnosis is important in this disease because treatment prevents further damage to the brain and liver.

- **Hallervorden Spatz Disease:**

This is also a rare, inherited progressive disease that begins in late childhood. Hallervorden Spatz Disease happens when too much iron collects in certain parts of the brain. There is no treatment for this disease.

- **Olivopontocerebellar Degeneration**:

This is an uncommon disorder where people have a hard time with balance and walking, often called Ataxia. People may have an action or sustention tremor, but do not have rigidity or bradykinesia.

The disorder results from a deterioration of the nervous system and does not respond to antiparkinson drugs.

- **Huntington's Disease:**

This is an inherited disease which usually begins early in middle life. People with this disease have involuntary movements (dyskinesias, chorea) that are associated with changes in behavior, personality, and mood.

The chorea (which resembles the involuntary movements caused by Levodopa) may happen before, during, or after the mental changes.

Once the disease is fully developed, it is easily distinguished from PD. However, the symptoms of a childhood form of Huntington's disease may resemble PD. Levodopa usually worsens the symptoms of Huntington's disease.

- **Dystonia:**

This is an inherited disease that begins in childhood and is progressive. People with this disease develop unusual postures of the head and neck, arms and legs.

This is called Generalized Dystonia. Another type of this disease is Segmental Dystonia. It develops in adulthood and involves only one part of the body, e.g. the head and neck.

- **Brain Tumors:**

Tumors of the brain that are close to the substantia nigra or the striatum may put local pressure on these parts of the brain. This local pressure may then result in the appearance of symptoms that look like PD.

A CT (CAT scan) or NMR (nuclear magnetic resonance scan) of the brain will exclude the possibility of a brain tumor as the cause of the Parkinsonian symptoms.

What is Early-Onset Parkinson's?

Early-Onset Parkinson's (also called Young-Onset Parkinson's or YOPD) is when symptoms of the disease appear before the age of 40. This happens to about 1 in 7 people with the disease.

Studies have shown that early-onset PD is not a lot different from the late-onset form. There are few differences though, that are listed below.

- levodopa therapy works but it is associated with on-off fluctuations and dyskinesias relatively early on in the disease

- the disease may progress more slowly than classic PD

- most people with early-onset PD have mostly rigid, akinetic (without movement) forms of the disease

- tremor is often a more prominent early symptom in early-onset PD than later-onset PD

- dystonia (abnormal PD muscle spasms) may show up earlier in early-onset PD than in later-onset

- dementia is rare in people with early-onset PD

- depression may occur more often and earlier on in the disease compared to people with later-onset PD

Do People With Early-Onset Parkinson's Have a Different Life Expectancy Than Those Who Are Diagnosed Later in Life?

The life expectancy of someone with early-onset PD is not affected by the disease, just like it is not affected by classic idiopathic PD.

There is evidence that the progression of the disease is slower in early-onset PD. This is because in younger people, tremor is usually predominant and its presence often means a slower progression of the disease.

Is the Chance of a Normal Life Less Likely for Someone Who has Been Diagnosed With PD Later in Life?

No, the chance of having a normal life does not have to be reduced if you are diagnosed later in life. Again, everybody's different and your symptoms may progress faster or slower than the average person with PD.

I had a great uncle who was diagnosed with Parkinson's in his late 70's and he lived for many years before his symptoms became debilitating.

Can Parkinson's Be Cured?

Well, we would certainly like to think so! Researchers are still working hard to find a cure and though they have not found one yet, they have made a lot of progress.

There is very real hope that the causes, whether genetic or environmental, will be figured out and the exact effects of these causes on how the brain works will be understood.

Even though there is currently no cure for Parkinson's disease, by identifying individual symptoms and determining the right kind of treatment, most people with the disease can live enjoyable, fulfilling lives.

SIGNS AND SYMPTOMS

What Are the Most Common Symptoms?

Symptoms of PD vary from person to person and not everyone is affected by all of them. In some people, the disease progresses quickly; in others it does not.

Here are the most common primary symptoms of Parkinson's disease:

Tremor:

In the early stages of the disease, about 70% of people experience a slight tremor in the hand or foot on one side of the body, or sometimes in the jaw or face. It looks like a 'beating' movement and is regular (4-6 beats per second).

Because tremor usually appears when the muscles are relaxed, it's called "resting tremor". This means that the affected body part trembles when it is at rest and not doing work and often stops when you start using (or working) that part of the body.

The tremor often spreads to the other side of the body as the disease progresses, but will remain most obvious on the side of the body where it first started.

A few more points on tremors include:

- usually occur at rest, may occur at any time
- may become severe enough to interfere with activities
- may be worse when tired, excited, or stressed
- finger-thumb rubbing (*pill-rolling tremor) may be present

*("pill-rolling" is seen especially in the hands; this is fairly unique to Parkinson's disease. The term refers to the motion that a pharmacist uses to align a handful of pills before placing them in a bottle or, possibly, the motion used to roll a marble between the thumb and forefinger. Eventually the tremor becomes more generalized.)

Rigidity:

Basically this means stiffness or inflexibility of the muscles. Normally muscles contract when they move, and then relax when they are at rest. In rigidity, the muscle tone of an affected body part is stiff.

Rigidity can result in a decreased range of motion. For example a person may not swing his or her arms when walking. Rigidity can also cause pain and cramps at the muscle site.

Bradykinesia:

Bradykinesia is a slowing of voluntary movement. In addition to slow movements, a person with bradykinesia will likely also have incompleteness of movement, difficulty in initiating movements, and arrests of ongoing movement.

The person may begin to walk with short, shuffling steps (festination), which, combined with other symptoms such as loss of balance, increases the incidence of falls.

They may also experience difficulty making turns or abrupt movements. They may go through periods of "freezing", which is when the person is stuck and finds it difficult to stop or start walking.

Bradykinesia and rigidity can occur in the facial muscles, causing a "mask-like" expression with little or no movement of the face. The slowness and incompleteness of movement can also affect speaking and swallowing.

Here is a list of some secondary symptoms of Parkinson's disease:

- **Speech/Voice Changes:**

    - slow speech

    - low-volume voice

    - monotone

    - difficulty speaking

- **Changes in Facial Expression:**

    - reduced ability to show facial expressions

    - "mask" appearance to face

- staring

- may be unable to close mouth

- reduced rate of blinking

- **Loss of Fine Motor Skills:**

  - difficulty writing, may be small and illegible (called micrographia)
  - difficulty eating

  - difficulty with any activity that requires small movements

  - movement is slow and uncontrolled

- **Difficulty swallowing**

- **Drooling**

- **Pain, including muscle aches and pains (myalgia)**

- **Dementia or confusion**

- **Sleep disturbances**

- **A variety of gastrointestinal symptoms, mainly constipation**

- **Skin problems**

- **Depression**

- **Fear, stress or anxiety**

- **Memory difficulties and slowed thinking**

- **Sexual difficulties**

- **Urinary problems**

- **Fatigue and/or loss of energy**

- **Unstable, stooped, or slumped-over posture**

What Are the Most Significant Signs to Look For to Determine if Someone Has Parkinson's?

In 50 to 80 percent of people with Parkinson's, the condition starts with the subtle so-called "pill-rolling" tremor of one hand. This is very typical (and was the first sign my mom had).

The uncontrollable tremor looks like the fingers are rolling a pill or a marble continuously. This is severe at rest and decreases during movement, and isn't there when the person is asleep.

Emotional stress, tension, and being tired make the tremor worse. Your hands, arms and legs are often affected, in that order.

In some people, there is no tremor, and rigidity of the muscles is present. The face becomes mask-like, expressionless, with less blinking and with mouth open.

Are There People Who Have Had All Their Symptoms Disappear?

We are not aware of anybody who has had all of their symptoms disappear without medications. With medications however, the main symptoms can disappear. Everybody experiences different success with medications but initially, you should experience the disappearance of the main symptoms of PD.

Mom has found her symptoms to disappear completely while at big parties like her wedding and her retirement party. These nights you could have sworn by looking at her that she didn't even have Parkinson's. Of course this is temporary but it does say something about how much your mood can affect your symptoms.

Why not throw yourself a party? Celebrate! Surely you can find a reason to have people over to the house for a get-together? You might be amazed at how much hanging out with people you love and who love you can help your symptoms disappear....

What Parts of the Body Are Affected?

The simplest answer is all the parts of the body. Well, that's what it may feel like sometimes, Mom says.

The brain is the first part of the body that is affected in a person with Parkinson's. As mentioned before, certain nerve cells in the small part of the brain called the "substantia nigra" start to degenerate and when they do a chemical messenger in the brain called dopamine is lost.

The substantia nigra has important connections with motor centers (brain centers that control movement) and so it plays a very important role in how we move. The chemical messenger dopamine is used by the substantia nigra so when dopamine is lost, messages to motor centers in the body can't go through. This results in mobility problems for people with Parkinson's.

Because dopamine is so important in the control of muscles, when it is lost the muscles act differently. Sometimes they tighten up, becoming stiff and rigid. In addition, movement becomes slow, problems develop with one's walking and posture and balance is also affected.

Parkinson's also affects the body temperature control system, digestive system, sexual function, and bladder control. Not all people with Parkinson's would necessarily experience difficulties with all of these however.

How Does Parkinson's Affect Behaviour?

Although everyone is different, Parkinson's can and probably will affect your personality which will then affect your behaviour.

As in my mom's case, though she was a pretty positive person to begin with, she isn't always able to be that way as much anymore (though I must admit she does a pretty good job at being positive most of the time). Obviously then, if a person with Parkinson's was not very positive to begin with, he or she would probably have an even harder time with the disease.

Another change in her behaviour is her lack of confidence. This has probably come gradually as she has lost to her ability to do some of the things she used to be able to.

Self-esteem can also be greatly affected by Parkinson's especially if you were lacking in this department before you got the disease. If you are at all self-conscious you may have a hard time being in public as you experience side effects of the disease like excessive shaking or moving of arms or legs.

How Does Parkinson's Affect a Person Psychologically?

Psychologically speaking, only a small amount of people with Parkinson's (about 15 to 20 percent) develop dementia which is an intellectual decline and loss of memory.

Many people with Parkinson's complain of problems like absent-mindedness, slowness of thinking and difficulty with mentally challenging tasks. However, not everyone with Parkinson's notice changes in their cognitive abilities (e.g. your ability to think).

My mom said she really noticed her inability to stay focussed on the task at hand very early on. She said she often felt like a "scatterbrain". This can be a result of Parkinson's medication, which controls production of dopamine, and may affect a person's ability to concentrate.

Now, sixteen years later, she notices from time to time she will say a word in a sentence that has absolutely nothing to do with what she is talking about. She's not sure why this happens, but figures it must have something to do with the disease.

Hallucinations, paranoia, and delusions are all possible side effects of Parkinson's disease medications. Switching to different Parkinson's disease medication can sometimes control these.

A hallucination occurs when you think something is present when it isn't. For example, you may hear a voice but no one is there. The hallucinations are not frightening and the Parkinsonian is well aware they are not real. If the drugs are working well, you may choose to live with this side effect.

An example of paranoia is when you think someone is following you when they are not. Delusion is when you are convinced something is true, despite clear evidence proving that it is not.

Parkinsonians may also suffer from nightmares and vivid dreams that are not a result of the Parkinson's but instead, the side effects of medications.

In order to deal with any previous psychological "challenges", the first step is to address any other medical conditions that could produce hallucinations, delusions, or paranoia.

Your doctor will check for things like imbalance of chemicals, possibly kidney, liver or lung function, as well as check for certain infections since these problems could cause mental disturbances.

Other medications that you may be using, including over-the-counter medicines, could also be responsible for these problems. Make sure you tell your doctor about all medications, including herbal therapies, that you are taking.

Some people may not be able to tolerate changes in their Parkinson's disease medications without increasing their symptoms. In these cases, it may be necessary to treat the mental disturbances with anti-psychotic medicines.

Unfortunately, some anti-psychotic medicines can worsen Parkinson's disease. There are alternatives though, and your doctor will be able to help you find them if you need to.

If you are experiencing any of the previously mentioned mental disturbances, talk to your doctor right away. There is likely a treatment that will make you feel better.

How Does Parkinson's Affect a Person's Emotions?

Parkinson's is a neurological, not a mental, disorder. In most cases, it slows the body, not the mind. However, when brain cells are affected by medication, you should expect some emotional changes.

Depression is a huge part of Parkinson's. Many people with the disease are affected by this. Paranoia, fear, and anxiety are also things that can be experienced by people who have the disease. My mom wonders if maybe these things come from losing your sense of confidence in things like walking and everyday activities.

Both anxiety and depression are very common among people with Parkinson's and may occur due to serotonin imbalance, a side effect of certain medications.

This may eventually lead to loss of memory. Anxiety and depression are difficult to diagnose in patients with Parkinson's because the symptoms are similar to those of the disease.

How Does Parkinson's Affect a Person's Social Life?

Socially speaking, it can be difficult for a person with Parkinson's because others may look at them as though they are, as my mom says, some sort of "freak" with all the involuntary moving (like the dyskinesia) that they're doing.

In reality, most people probably don't look at people with Parkinson's as freaks but it's easy to feel that way when you have the disease.

As the disease progresses, it can be hard to be in public sometimes. For instance, when my mom experiences a sudden shutdown of her body she'll often have troubles walking through doorways. This can attract a lot of attention from others and can be very emotionally disturbing to any person with Parkinson's.

Also, when eating out, it can be hard at times for the person with Parkinson's because it's often hard to hold onto cutlery. Several times, my mom has been embarrassed and upset because she can't stop dropping things at the dinner table. Even amongst friends, she at times finds it very hard emotionally to do things like this.

Finally, it can sometimes be hard on your social life if you have a partner (for example, a husband or wife) and if you can no longer do the things the way you used to (like going dancing).

Can Parkinson's Turn Into Alzheimer's Disease?

At this point, researchers are still trying to figure this out. Some believe that Parkinson's and Alzheimer's disease cannot exist at the same time but others believe they can.

In the early stages of Parkinson's, dementia is somewhat different from the dementia seen in Alzheimer's disease. In Parkinson's the dementia can be seen as being forgetful, having a hard time making decisions, planning, reasoning, having slow thought processes, etc. In Alzheimer's there is a great loss of memory and intellectual abilities.

In the later stages, the dementia in Parkinson's can be as severe as that seen in Alzheimer's disease. About 20 to 25% of people in the later stages of Parkinson's develop dementia severe enough to interfere with day-to-day functioning. This is about 10-15% higher than the general population at the same age. Unfortunately, though, it's impossible to predict which people with Parkinson's will develop this problem.

Does Parkinson's Lead to Early Dementia?

As mentioned in the previous question, it is thought that about 20 to 25% of people in the later stages of Parkinson's develop dementia severe enough to interfere with day-to-day functioning. This is about 10-15% higher than the general population at the same age.

Unfortunately, though, it's impossible to predict which people with Parkinson's will develop this problem.

Although people with Parkinson's are at a slightly increased risk for developing dementia, most people won't have problems with this.

When a person with PD begins to show signs of dementia, it is important that a careful search is made for treatable conditions. Two possible causes of dementia in PD that can be treated include medications and depression.

Many antiparkinsonian medications interfere with thinking and memory, especially drugs in the class known as anticholinergics, including Artane and Cogentin. All antiparkinsonian medications have the potential to cause confusion.

Depression is a common problem in PD and may seem like dementia with its symptoms of poor concentration, thinking and memory. These symptoms do go away, though, as soon as the depression is treated.

Do Long Term PD Patients Develop Memory and Reasoning Problems or Could Meds for PD Cause This?

Yes, long term Parkinson's patients do develop memory and reasoning problems related to dementia about 15 to 20 percent of the time. Sometimes this can happen at middle-age but generally speaking these problems happen when you get older.

About 20% of people taking levodopa may experience side effects of confusion, delusions, and hallucinations but these symptoms occur more frequently in older people with a later onset of the disease.

Does Parkinson's Cause Depression Or Is It a Side Effect of the Drugs?

Well, it can be both. Depression is common in people with Parkinson's and can happen as a result of the disease and/or because of the side effects of the drugs taken for the disease. For most people with Parkinson's disease, depression can be controlled.

Depression can actually increase the physical effects of Parkinson's disease and possibly cause a progression of the disease. If you experience five or more of the following symptoms for longer than two weeks at a time, you should contact your doctor.

- Depressed mood

- An inability to find pleasure in things that were once pleasurable

- Sleep disturbances (inability to sleep or sleeping excessively)

- Change in appetite

- Fatigue

- Altered level of activity

- Difficulty with concentration

- Low self-esteem

- Thoughts of death

Depression may be treated with psychological therapy, as well as with medications. People seem to do better when they receive both psychological and drug treatments.

*NOTE: Make sure you check with your pharmacist about taking any new medications (like antidepressants) as there may be some that may not be compatible with your PD medications.

There are many anti-depressant medications available, each with its own advantages and disadvantages. Your doctor will know which ones are best for you.

Most people with Parkinson's disease should not take Ascendin (amoxipine) because this medication could temporarily worsen the Parkinson's disease symptoms.

Psychological therapy can help people with Parkinson's disease regain their sense of self-worth even though they may not be able to do as much anymore.

It also can help the person maintain good relationships with caregivers and family members, despite having to depend on them more.

Is it Normal for Someone with Parkinson's to Experience Anxiety?

Yes! It is absolutely normal for someone with Parkinson's to experience anxiety. There are so many reasons why you could feel anxious. The minute you get diagnosed with this disease, there are things to be anxious about.

People with PD may experience anxiety in various ways including feeling fearful, worrying constantly to the point where it can't be controlled, and having various physical symptoms such as muscle tension, palpitations, sweating, and shortness of breath.

In order to be treated, you need to find the source of the anxiety. Anxiety can often be the main symptom of depression so it's important to find out if you are suffering from depression so you can be treated for that.

Anxiety often accompanies the "off" periods when a person with PD is experiencing immobility. The anxiety that a person can have with the off period can be severe and the anxiety and immobility feed off each other, making both worse over time.

To help manage this anxiety, you first have to be diagnosed and then you should have your antiparkinson medications reviewed and adjusted to minimize your off periods.

It's important to be educated about the link between anxiety and the off period and reassured that even a long off period will eventually resolve.

If you have PD and experience long off periods, you may find that taking 0.5 mg of lorazepam as needed under your tongue may make your anxiety more manageable. Talk to your doctor if you think you may need or want this.

Having PD is not much different than having any other disease in that oftentimes being proactive and finding out more about it can help.

Is Stress a Factor in Making Symptoms Worse?

YES! Stress can have a very negative impact on the symptoms of Parkinson's disease, so it's important to focus on managing the stress in your daily life and finding some relaxation.

Stress and chronic illness go hand in hand. Stress comes from a variety of different sources that can be physical, as well as emotional.

Stress can come from daily life tasks, events, problems, fatigue, as well as anxiety and frustration with having to deal with the limitations and life adjustments that Parkinson's disease often creates.

The important thing to be aware of, however, is that stress can worsen Parkinson's disease symptoms, especially tremor and mobility. Therefore, it is important to focus on stress management and relaxation in your daily life.

The following are some stress management techniques you may want to incorporate into your life. Not all techniques work for everyone. You have to experiment a little to find something that works for you. Try more than one technique, and then use it often. Remember that the key to successful stress management is practice.

Deep Breathing:

Take slow, deep breaths from your diaphragm. Breathe in through your nose and out through your mouth. Count to five as you breathe in and five as you breathe out. Do this several times until you begin to feel more relaxed.

Progressive Relaxation:

Get in a comfortable position, close your eyes and slowly focus on relaxing different parts of your body, one at a time. Start from your head and work down to your feet. There are many different relaxation tapes out there that can guide you.

Relaxation Tapes/CDs/Books:

There are many different relaxation materials available in bookstores and over the internet. Music stores usually have a section on relaxation. You may have to experiment a little to find something that works for you.

Meditation:

There are many good books and tapes on this topic. You may also be able to find classes that are offered in your community.

Massage:

Massage can be very helpful in relieving muscle tightness, but it is also extremely relaxing to body and mind. Mom loves this and gets a good half hour to an hour massage as often as she can.

Is Difficulty Sleeping a Symptom or Side Effect of the Drugs?

Having difficulties sleeping are common in people with PD and can be both a symptom of the disease and a side effect of the drugs.

The drugs Sinemet and sometimes Eldepryl can interfere with sleep.

Taking your medications at different times may help your difficulties with sleep, but there is no magic formula that works for everyone.

It may take some time to figure out when the best times to take your medications are, and whether or not you need to change the dosage before bedtime. Your doctor can help you with this.

Does Parkinson's Have an Affect on Blood Pressure?

People with Parkinson's may experience low blood pressure due to the medications that are taken for the disease.

Some people with PD also have a history of high blood pressure (hypertension) and are already taking medication to lower it. Adding an antiparkinson drug can lower the blood pressure even further, resulting in dizziness or fainting. In this case, the medication for high blood pressure can often be reduced or stopped.

There a few things that you can do if your blood pressure is low because of your PD medications:

- Avoid standing, especially after exercise, since blood will pool in your legs. If standing at the sink or a workbench, keep your feet moving a little.

- Avoid very hot baths or showers, and always sit down to towel off.

- Get up slowly from the lying position, and avoid getting up from a meal too quickly.

- Make sure that you drink plenty of fluids and use extra salt.

Does Parkinson's Disease Affect the Heart Valves?

No, not exactly. It's not the disease which affects the heart valves, but possibly a medication used in treating the disease.

There's a drug named Pergolide which is used to treat tremors in Parkinson's disease that may be responsible for heart damage.

Researchers say that there is enough evidence to recommend that anyone with heart problems not take Pergolide, which is sold as Permax and has been used since 1989 to treat the tremors and restless leg syndrome of people with Parkinson's disease.

More research needs to be done about this condition but, in the meantime, researchers have stated that "Pergolide should be discontinued if valvular disease is detected and no other cause identified."

How Does Parkinson's Affect Gait?

Some people with Parkinson's have difficulty starting to walk. They have problems lifting their foot in order to start walking and may take a few small and uneasy steps before walking at a steady pace.

While they are walking, they stop swinging their arms. They will also shuffle (a bunch of small, short steps) their feet and walk with their body weight on the front part of their feet.

Festinant gait is when a person starts taking small short shuffling steps that become faster and faster. What sometimes happens is that the shuffling becomes so fast that he/she falls forward or runs into something.

Sometimes the same happens only backwards. There was a time when my mom had problems with this. For what seemed like no reason at all, she would just start shuffling backwards. We laughed at it to help her be less anxious, and would say "Hey Mom, you need to switch gears, you're in reverse!"

You need to be careful as the caregiver if and when you see someone with Parkinson's shuffling because this can often lead to falls. About one-third of people with Parkinson's disease fall relatively frequently. People with Parkinson's lose their ability to regain their balance when they start to fall so it is important to stay near them if they're having walking difficulties.

Something called freezing can also happen when a person with Parkinson's is walking. This often happens in doorways, and basically makes it impossible for the person to move. It is like their feet are glued to the ground.

What is Dyskinesia and What Can be Done to Help Stop It?

Dyskinesia is basically abnormal, involuntary movements. It is caused by too much dopamine in your system. Once the effects of your medication start to wear off, you take higher doses and this causes the excess of dopamine.

Some studies say that the drug amantadine may be useful for the management of levodopa-induced dyskinesia, but it is not a long term solution for it.

One simple way that my mom has found to help stop her dyskinesia is to go for a brisk walk. She says that doing any kind of, as she says "purposeful activity" helps make the dyskinesia go away.

Does Parkinson's Cause Back Pain and Pain in Other Areas?

Yes, Parkinson's can cause pain in your back and other areas. First you should figure out whether there may be other causes for your pain, though, such as arthritis. Talk to your doctor.

You often get back pain because of the strain placed on your back from the stooped posture which is common in people with Parkinson's.

If you do experience pain in your limbs or back area, it will probably appear along with other more typical symptoms of PD, like tremor and slowness.

If your pain does accompany your other PD symptoms, and improves when these are improved by PD medications, then you should talk to your doctor about adjusting the dosage or frequency of your PD medications. The treatment for pain caused by PD is most often the same as the treatment for motor symptoms of PD.

Another reason you might experience pain is because of leg cramping. Pain caused by cramping can be a sign of a recent increase in activity, and in this case the pain usually goes away after the exercise becomes more routine.

Pain can also occur as your medications are wearing off.

If the typical anti-cramping suggestions like exercise, massage, the application of heat, etc., don't relieve the cramping well enough, you might need to try anti-cramping medications. Talk to your doctor about it and he or she can help you figure out what might work for you the best.

For more information on the different kinds of pain that may accompany PD and ways to treat them, check out the **BONUS: Pain and Parkinson's Disease: Answers to Common Questions (p.119).**

Does Parkinson's Affect Vision?

Yes, Parkinson's can affect your vision. Problems with vision can occur as a symptom of the disease and/or as a side effect of medications.

You might find that your "upgaze", or ability to look up at things like signs that are above you, is not very good. Some people also have difficulties in adjusting their eyes to changing light levels and find it hard to see at night.

Blurry vision can be a side effect of anticholinergics (drugs used to control tremor). It can also be caused by the lack of blinking that occurs as a side effect of the disease.

What is Myerson's Sign?

If you were to tap on the glabella (the area between your eyebrows, just above your nose) of someone who does not have Parkinson's, at first they would start blinking, but then they would stop even if you kept tapping.

Sometimes in Parkinson's patients, if you were to tap on this same spot, they would just keep on blinking, and not be able to stop. This is what's called "Myerson's Sign".

What is Dysarthria and How Does it Affect a Person With Parkinson's?

Dysarthria means difficulty speaking. About half of all people with Parkinson's have problems with speech which can include difficulties with volume, phrasing, rhythm, and clarity.

Here are some of the typical problems that people with PD may have with speech:

- slurring words often

- a soft and quiet voice (so quiet you sometimes can't even hear it)

- sudden pauses or long breaks in the middle of a sentence while trying to remember a word or thought

- a dull tone of voice, with no energy or rhythm

- a hurried way of speaking that sometimes seems like a stutter

- slow speech patterns, with repeated sounds and stops

Ask your doctor to see what's best for you, but being that this can be a severely limiting symptom of Parkinson's disease, seeing a speech pathologist may be your best option.

Is There a Skin Condition Associated With Parkinson's?

If you have Parkinson's disease, it is common for the skin on your face to become very oily, especially on the forehead and at the sides of the nose (this is known as Seborrhea). The scalp may become oily too, resulting in dandruff. In other cases, the skin can become very dry.

These problems are also the result of an autonomic nervous system that's not working properly. Standard treatments for skin problems help. Sweating a lot is another common symptom, and is usually controllable with medications used for Parkinson's disease.

There is also an odd skin condition (called "livedo reticularis") that is a side effect of the drug Symmetrel (variety of amantadine used for treating dyskinesia).

The signs of this condition are purple blotches on your thighs and forearms, and swelling in your feet. These markings sometimes stay on your body even after you stop taking the medication that caused them.

Is Constipation Caused by Parkinson's or the Medications You Take for Parkinson's?

Constipation is a common complaint for people with PD. It is a symptom of the disease but can be worsened by medications.

Many factors other than medications can contribute to constipation. Stress, depression, poor eating habits, lack of exercise, and not drinking enough fluids can all take their toll on your body.

Instead of simply trying to manage this problem, you should also try to prevent it.

Here are a few things that might help:

- Increase your daily fluid intake, especially in hot weather. Try drinking at least six cups of liquid daily.

- Older people may not be able to tolerate large amounts of raw fruit and vegetables, but can usually manage dried fruits, hot prune juice, canned fruits, and soft cooked vegetables, all of which may help.

- Adding a high-fibre cereal to your diet is important, but it should be started slowly and in small amounts. Large amounts can cause stomach cramps and excess gas, particularly in people who cannot exercise.

- Exercising regularly is very important.

- Stool softeners, bulk laxatives, and bowel stimulants are the main kinds of laxatives available over-the-counter. If changing your diet doesn't work, you can try any one of these.

TREATMENT AND MEDICATION

How Do You Treat Parkinson's?

In order to treat Parkinson's you will need access to most, if not all of the following people:

- neurologist (your doctor will refer you to one who will decide on your treatment plan)

- occupational and/or physical therapist (if you need to relearn how to dress, shower, eat and perform other everyday tasks smoothly)

- massage therapist

- counsellor (to help you adjust to your diagnosis and the changes it means for your lifestyle)

- social worker, psychologist, or psychiatrist (for depression)

- speech therapist (if you need help with communication)

- registered dietician

Generally speaking, the treatment for Parkinson's disease is designed to:

- Maintain overall quality of life
- Improve mobility and function
- Reduce rigidity
- Reduce tremor
- Reverse slowed movements
- Improve posture, gait, balance, speech, and writing skills
- Maintain mental sharpness

Most people with Parkinson's disease can be treated using prescribed medications. Check out **Question #57:"What are the latest drug treatments for Parkinson's?" (p. 47)** to find out what kind of drugs your doctor might prescribe for you.

If you don't react well to medications, or if the medications stop working, you might be advised to have surgery.

Depending upon your needs, medical history, health, and symptoms, one of the following procedures may be considered:

- **Deep brain stimulation**

- **Pallidotomy**

- **Thalamotomy**

- **Gamma knife**

These procedures are all explained in the answer to **Question #77: "Is there an operation for people with PD which can improve their quality of life?" (p. 71)**

There are many other procedures being researched. **Questions # 79: "What is fetal cell transplantation?" on p. 76** and **#80: "How can stem cells help someone with PD?" on p. 77** discuss some of the most recent developments in treating PD.

Alternative therapy may also be used, see answer to **Question #73: "What alternative treatments are available for Parkinson's?" (p. 65)**

What Medications Do You Start With?

Your doctor will decide which medications and proper dosages are best for you. He or she will probably monitor you closely for the first while to see if the medications and dosages are working right for you.

In my mom's case, after she was diagnosed she started on the two main drugs used to treat Parkinson's; Sinemet (levodopa-carbidopa) and Selegilene (also known as Deprenyl).

The Sinemet was prescribed to help keep the dopamine levels in her brain from falling too much and the Selegilene was prescribed to help slow the progression of the disease, and help the Sinemet work more effectively.

Now, sixteen years later, Mom is on a very similar treatment plan as the one she was on when she was diagnosed. She now takes the Controlled-Release (CR) version of Sinemet and takes the drug Mirapex.

She has also had to increase the dosages of these meds over the years, as her body over time has become used to them and requires more to do the same job.

How Can a Person With PD Get the Most Out of Their Medications?

Here are a few things you might like to try to increase the effectiveness of your medications:

- Take the medication as prescribed by your doctor. Make sure you understand the expected benefit and potential early side effects of a drug before you leave the doctor's office. Remember that he (or she) probably has more clinical experience in treating people with Parkinson's disease than anyone else who is likely to give you advice.

- All side effects of antiparkinson drugs are reversible by lowering or stopping the dosage.

- Do not increase or suddenly stop any of your drugs without checking it out with your doctor first.

- Take medications with food as taking them on an empty stomach often leads to increased side effects. Note: some meds need to be taken on an empty stomach to get the most benefits from them; check with your doctor first.

- Another tip Mom had was to avoid eating large amounts of protein at any time. She has found that eating too much protein really reduces the effectiveness of her meds.

How Do You Know If You Are Getting the Most Out of Your Medications?
(How Much "Off" Time is Reasonable?)

Though you may not always be able to achieve it, you should be aiming for as little "off" or "down" time as possible (e.g. time when you are basically having to stay put in one place for a period of time because your medications have worn off).

Some people with Parkinson's will find that after they take their meds there is a period of time before they kick in. This is true for my mom. She usually expects to have to wait up to 45 minutes (usually less than this) after she takes her medications for them to start working and her to have "on" time (or in her words, for her to "have wheels").

Her way of telling whether or not she is getting the most out of her meds is to see how much time each day she spends in "off" mode. For her, if she has to wait more than an hour for her meds to kick in, or has more than four hours in one day in this down time, she knows she needs to talk to her doctor about possibly changing the dosage and/or timing of her medications.

One thing that has helped the effectiveness of her meds is being able to take them on an empty stomach. This wasn't possible for her in the beginning because she got nauseous all the time (a common side effect of the drugs) but after her body got used to it, she was able to switch the timing of taking her meds.

Mom says the good thing about having less food in your stomach is that the meds work better but sometimes it can seem they are working too well because you get more of the side effect dyskinesia. You might have to experiment a bit with the timing of your meals and meds in order to find what's best for you.

One tip Mom had for helping your medications work better is to avoid sitting in one place for long lengths of time. If you have to sit anywhere for over an hour at a time, try to get up every hour and do some stretching or moving around to keep your muscles from stiffening up too much.

Mom says regardless of when she last took her medications, sitting in one spot for a long time can really make it hard to get moving again.

What Are the Latest Drug Treatments for Parkinson's?

There have been some amazing changes over the past decade in treating Parkinson's disease. Researchers have made new medications and are able to understand how to use them better than before. This has really helped to improve the quality of life in people with the disease.

There are two general ways to treat Parkinson's disease with medication. The first is to try and slow the loss of dopamine in the brain and the second is to try and improve the symptoms of Parkinson's disease by other means.

Most people with Parkinson's disease can be treated well enough with medications that help get rid of their symptoms.

Remember that you have the right and responsibility to know what medications are being prescribed for you. The more you know about your medications and how they work, the easier it will be for you to control your symptoms.

The following is a list of drugs that may be prescribed to you by your doctor. Don't be afraid to talk with him or her about your treatment plan. You are in this disease together.

Five classes of drugs used to treat symptoms of PD:

Dopaminergic Agents:

- **Levodopa**

Levodopa (also called L-dopa) is converted in the brain into dopamine, the same chemical created by substantia nigra cells and used to control movement.

Levodopa was introduced as a PD therapy in the 1960s, and remains the most effective therapy for motor symptoms. It lessens and helps to control all the major motor symptoms of PD, including bradykinesia, which is generally the most disabling part of the disease.

- **Sinemet (levodopa/carbidopa)**

Sinemet is made up of levodopa and another drug called carbidopa. Levodopa enters the brain and is converted to dopamine while carbidopa prevents or lessens many of the side effects of levodopa, such as nausea, vomiting, and occasional heart rhythm disturbances.

There are two forms of Sinemet, controlled-release or immediate-release Sinemet. Controlled-release (CR) Sinemet and immediate-release Sinemet are equally effective in treating the symptoms of Parkinson's disease, but some people prefer the controlled release version. Ask your doctor which approach is best for you.

Even though Sinemet is the most effective medication and has the least short-term side effects, there is also a high risk of long-term side effects, such as involuntary movements (dyskinesia).

If you use levodopa on a long-term basis, you may experience restlessness, confusion, or abnormal movements.

Changes in the amount or timing of the dose will usually prevent these side effects, but most experts now recommend alternatives to Sinemet, like dopamine agonists, and use Sinemet only when the alternatives fail to work the way you'd like them to.

- **Dopamine Agonists**

Dopamine Agonists are drugs that imitate what levodopa does in the brain.

Even though they are not quite as effective as levodopa, they really help the symptoms and delay the start of mobility problems.

There are a variety of dopamine agonists that are available:

- Apomorphine (Apokyn)

- Bromocriptine (Parlodel)

- Pergolide (Permax)

- Pramipexole (Mirapex)

- Ropinirole (Requip)

- Cabergoline (Not approved in the US as of late 2004)

- Lisuride (Not approved in the US as of late 2004)

Requip and Mirapex are newer medications, and are safer and more effective than the older drugs, Parlodel and Permax.

Newer dopamine agonists like Requip are often the first choice of treatment for Parkinson's disease because they don't have the same risks of long-term problems as levodopa therapy does.

COMT Inhibitors:

- Entacapone (Comtan)

- Tolcapone (Tasmar)

COMT inhibitors help make a dose of levodopa work longer by preventing it from breaking down.

Both Entacapone (Comtan) and Tolcapone (Tasmar) have been shown to decrease the amount of "off" time (the period of time when PD symptoms are present). off or down /

Tolcapone is more effective than Entacapone, reducing off time in clinical trials by 2-3 hours, versus 1 to 2 hours for Entacapone.

By taking these drugs, you are usually able to reduce your levodopa dose by 20%-25%.

MAO-B Inhibitors:

- Rasagiline

- Selegiline (Eldepryl/Deprenyl)

On May 16 2006, the FDA approved Rasagiline in 0.5 and 1 mg tablets (Azilect, made by Teva Pharmaceutical Industries, Inc) for use as initial monotherapy in the treatment of early Parkinson's disease and for use in addition to levodopa therapy for people who have moderate to advanced PD.

Results from one 26-week study of patients with early Parkinson's disease showed that rasagiline monotherapy significantly reduced the decline in a person's ability to think, their ability to perform activities of daily living, and their motor function.

Selegiline, Eldepryl and Deprenyl are all names for the same drug. They work by helping to conserve the amount of dopamine available by preventing the dopamine from being destroyed.

Though not all researchers have been able to agree on this one, there is some evidence that this drug may slow the progression of Parkinson's, especially early on in the disease.

This drug is well-tolerated by most people, so many experts recommend using it despite the controversies. Common side effects are nausea and vomiting.

Anticholinergics:

- Trihexyphenidyl (Artane)

- Benztropine

- Ethopropazine

Anticholinergics have a limited role in PD. They are mostly effective against tremor and rigidity, and their side effects may be greater, especially in older people.

Amantadine (Symmetrel):

Amantadine (Symmetrel) helps reduce the motor symptoms of PD (by increasing the amount of dopamine available for use in the brain) somewhat, but helps reduce dyskinesia even more.

Symmetrel may be helpful in treating people with mild Parkinson's disease, but it often causes significant side-effects including confusion and memory problems.

Is it Safe to Take Other Drugs While on PD Medication?

Most drugs are safe to take with antiparkinson drugs. There are a few drugs that need special attention though:

- One group of drugs known as dopamine antagonists (for example haloperidol (Haldol), rispiridone (Risperdal) and metoclopromide (Maxeran), prochlorperazine (Stemetil), chlorpromazine (Largacty and Zyprexa) should be avoided because they can worsen the symptoms of Parkinson's by blocking the action of dopamine in the brain.

  They are generally prescribed for nausea or psychiatric conditions. Check with your doctor or pharmacist if you are not sure whether you have been prescribed one of these.

- Demerol (often used to control postoperative pain) can cause confusion and hallucinations in people with PD and should be avoided.

- Always remember to talk to your doctor about any concerns you may have about drug interactions

Tips on Avoiding Interactions With Other Medications:

- Read all of your medication labels carefully.

- Make all health care providers aware of all the medications you are using.

- Know your drug and food allergies.

- Make a list of your medications and dosages. Eye drops, skin lotions and vitamins are considered medications and should be included on your list. Keep this with you and update when you need to.

- Review possible drug side effects. Most reactions will happen when a new drug is started, but not always. Some reactions may be delayed or might happen when a new medication is added.

- Use one pharmacy if possible. Try to fill all your prescriptions at the same pharmacy, so the pharmacist can monitor for interactions and provide proper dosing and refills.

What Are the Side Effects of Sinemet?

Sinemet is a Parkinson's disease drug that is a combination of levodopa and carbidopa. This combination reduces the harmful side effects caused by using levodopa over a long period of time.

Most people taking Sinemet experience side effects, but these may go away during treatment as your body adjusts to the medicine.

Here are some possible side effects that may occur and usually do not need medical attention: (yes, this list is long but remember that you won't have all these side effects)

- occasional involuntary movements (May include chewing, gnawing, twisting, tongue or mouth movements, head bobbing, or movements of the feet, hands, or shoulder. These may respond to a reduction in the dose.)

- loss of appetite

- darker colored urine, saliva and sweat (Urine may at first be reddish, then turn to nearly black after being exposed to air. Some bathroom cleaning products will produce a similar effect when in contact with urine containing this medicine. This is to be expected while taking this medicine.)

- dry mouth

- upset stomach (other medications such as Permax can cause this as well)

- headache

- dizziness (you may get dizzy when you stand up due to the drop in blood pressure; get up slowly over several minutes from sitting or lying position and be careful climbing stairs)

- abdominal pain

- change in taste (may cause a bitter taste, or a burning sensation on your tongue)

- increased sweating

- light headed (avoid driving, doing other tasks or activities where you need to be alert until you see how this medicine affects you)

- passing gas

- trouble sleeping (including nightmares)

- constipation

- diarrhoea

- hiccups

NOTE: If you find these side effects to continue or become too much trouble, talk to your doctor.

Other side effects not listed above may also occur in some people. If you notice any other effects, check with your doctor.

Here are some reasons not to take this medicine:

- If you have an allergy to carbidopa, levodopa, or any other part of the medicine.

- If you have any of the following conditions: Narrow-angle glaucoma, history of melanoma, unexplained skin spots.

- If you have taken a monoamine oxidase inhibitor (phenelzine, tranylcypromine, isocarboxazid) in the last 14 days.

If You Go Off Sinemet, How Will You Be Affected?

Do not stop taking Sinemet (a combination of carbidopa and levodopa) suddenly. It may take several weeks before you feel the full effects of this medicine. Stopping suddenly could make your condition much worse.

You should not suddenly stop taking this medicine unless your doctor tells you otherwise.

How Can Side Effects of PD Drugs Be Managed?

One of the major side effects of the antiparkinson medication Sinemet is nausea. Nausea is much less common with controlled-release Sinemet, which is absorbed more slowly than the regular Sinemet.

Dopamine agonists can cause nausea even in people who did not experience it with either kind of Sinemet. Building up your dose very slowly can help, even though you may be impatient to feel the improvement in your PD symptoms.

In Canada and other parts of the world there is a drug called domperidone (Motilium) which is used to prevent the nausea caused by antiparkinson drugs.

Some ways to control or relieve nausea are:

- Drink clear or ice-cold drinks. Drinks containing sugar may calm the stomach better than other liquids.

- Avoid orange and grapefruit juices because these are too acidic and may worsen nausea.

- Drink your drinks slowly.

- Drink liquids between meals instead of during them.

- Eat light, bland foods (such as saltine crackers or plain bread).

- Avoid fried, greasy or sweet food.

- Eat slowly.

- Eat smaller, more frequent meals throughout the day.

- Don't mix hot and cold foods.

- Eat foods that are cold or at room temperature to avoid getting nauseated from the smell of hot or warm foods.

- Rest after eating, keeping your head elevated. Activity may make your nausea worse and may lead to vomiting.

- Avoid brushing your teeth after eating.

- If you feel nauseated when you wake up in the morning, eat some crackers before getting out of bed or eat a high protein snack before going to bed (lean meat or cheese).

- Try to eat when you feel less nauseated.

*If these techniques don't seem to help your queasy stomach, ask your doctor for more ideas.

Another major side effect of antiparkinson drugs is dizziness. Dizziness occurs due to the fact that the drugs can lower your blood pressure. It may occur in the early stages of treatment, but it usually resolves over time. If it doesn't, talk to your doctor.

How Can You Prevent "Freezing"?

- count your steps as you walk (try marching or "left, right, left, right...)

- one great thing Mom discovered was music - try putting on a CD with some fast-paced music on to keep you going - even better, carry an MP3 player around with your favourite tunes on it so you can "plug in" anytime you need a lift **(read more about this in the Bonus questions).**

Let's face it, you may not always be able to prevent freezing. Here are some ways to help you out if you do:

- rock in place from foot to foot to get moving again

- have someone place their foot in front of you, or visualize something you need to step over

- try covering your eyes- this can "trick" your brain and allow you to walk straight ahead with no problems

- you may choose to simply wait after all, the freezing will pass

- if you are in a hurry you can slowly sink to your knees and crawl but obviously this is only practical at home

- walk very carefully backwards or sideways (this works very well for my mom)

What Can Be Done to Help Increase Mobility In People With PD?

The first step is to ask your doctor for an evaluation by a physical therapist. The therapist will make up a detailed evaluation with recommendations for your treatment.

Physical therapy cannot stop the disease, but it may help slow down the loss of mobility that comes with PD.

Physical therapists teach people with PD and their caregivers' exercises to increase mobility and techniques to deal with specific trouble areas such as freezing, getting in and out of bed, getting up from a sitting position, etc.

Physical therapy can help people who are in various stages of Parkinson's - from the recently diagnosed to those who have had Parkinson's for many years.

My mom has found physical therapy to be very helpful. She goes once a week. She also tries to get outside everyday to do some form of exercise. This is to help her keep her mobility for as long as possible (remember the statement; "use it or lose it!").

Getting outside also helps prevent depression which can often make you lose your motivation to do any exercise.

Something else that Mom has found helpful in increasing her mobility is massage therapy. She loves this and goes once a week (she'd go more if she could afford it).

How Can You Get Rid of the Tremors?

Tremors can be a real pain in the butt and though there's no way to prevent them, you can take steps to reduce them.

Stay away from stimulants like caffeine and amphetamines. Although small amounts of alcohol may reduce tremor, try not to drink large amounts of alcohol because it can make the tremors worse.

People with Parkinson's disease have had success with levodopa or other antiparkinson drugs.

There is also a surgical procedure called Deep brain stimulation (DBS) that can be used to treat tremors in people with Parkinson's (it also helps reduce rigidity, stiffness, slowed movement, and walking problems). You can read more about this procedure in the answer to **Question #77: "Is there an operation for people with PD which can improve their quality of life?" (p.71)**

At this point, the procedure is used only for people who have symptoms that can't be controlled well enough with medications.

What is the Patch and Will It Help With Tremors?

Researchers are developing a new way to deliver drugs for Parkinson's to the brain. The "Parkinson's Patch" gives a steady, uniform dosage of medication, which reduces the risk of side effects.

Rather than swallowing pills several times a day, people apply patches to their chest just once a day.

Doctors hope to learn whether this new delivery system can improve the motor symptoms of Parkinson's disease in a consistent, smooth fashion.

They hope the continuous delivery of drugs made possible by the patch technology will more closely imitate the brain's own actions.

UPDATE: The new patch form of drug has been recently approved in the US to treat people with early Parkinson's.

The once-daily Neupro patch contains a drug called rotigotine, which has not been sold before in the United States. The drug patch, made by Schwarz Pharma AG, is the first for the treatment of symptoms of Parkinson's disease.

Can Nicotine Help With Parkinson's?

It is known that most people with Parkinson's never (or only for a very short period) smoked cigarettes. This fact originally led researchers to the idea that something in nicotine helps to prevent PD. So far, however, no researcher has been able to figure out what in nicotine MAY have some protective aspect.

Researchers are now looking at ways of using nicotine to make some of the symptoms of PD not as bad.

In a few small studies, the people studied found some benefit to their PD symptoms while on a nicotine patch.

It is still too soon to tell whether or not nicotine is of any real benefit to people with PD. It will have to undergo many further studies before doctors can recommend this as a treatment for PD.

Researchers are also trying to make sure that these nicotine patches will not cause addiction to nicotine - similar to that seen in people who smoke.

How Can You Prevent Drooling?

People with PD don't have more saliva than people without PD, they just swallow less often. As a result of this, there ends up being an excess amount of saliva which then often results in drooling.

On October 1, 2006, the Centers for Medicare and Medicaid approved payment for the use of injections of Botulinum Toxin Type A (Botox) to help reduce drooling (also called sialorrhea).

Talk to your doctor if you are having problems with drooling as this may be an alternative for you if nothing else has worked.

Here are a few other suggestions which may help prevent drooling and possibly some embarrassing moments:

- suck on hard candy, lozenges or gum to control excess saliva (if you are not at risk of choking)

- use a straw when drinking to strengthen the muscles of the lips, mouth and throat

- try to keep your head up and your posture straight because stooping encourages drooling

- swallow first before you talk

- when you're not eating or talking, keep your mouth closed and your lips tight together (people with PD tend to let their jaw drop open which encourages drooling)

- breathe through your nose (this will help keep your mouth closed which will then help keep the saliva in your mouth)

- remind yourself to swallow to help prevent saliva build up

- you may try rubbing a strong smelling lip balm over your mouth to remind you to swallow

- try putting one or two drops of atropine eye drops (0.5%) under your tongue to reduce the amount of saliva- this works for some people but you should check with your doctor first

How Can You Help Dry Mouth?

- if you are not at risk of choking, suck on hard candies or chew gum to help keep your mouth wet/lubricated

- try not to eat too many dry foods like peanut butter, crackers and chips because they stick to the throat and dry out the mouth

- eat sour candy or fruit ice to help increase saliva and moisten your mouth

- add sauces to foods to make them softer and moister (ex. gravy, broth, sauce, or melted butter)

- take a drink after each bite of food to moisten your mouth and to help you swallow

- dunk or moisten breads, toast, cookies, or crackers in milk, tea, or coffee to soften them

- breath through your nose instead of your mouth

- keep hydrated, drinking lots of water (8 glasses a day will help) *Note: some people with Parkinson's disease who also have heart problems may need to limit their fluids, so be sure to follow your doctor's guidelines.

- if you smoke, try to cut down or even quit because this can be a major factor in drying out your mouth and causing gum problems

- try taking a cotton swab dipped in olive oil and rubbing it on the inside of your mouth and throat with it every hour or so

- don't use a commercial mouthwash because they often contain alcohol that can dry your mouth. Ask your doctor or dentist about alternative mouthwash products.

- limit caffeine (contained in coffee, tea, cola, and chocolate) as it may interfere with some of your medications and may actually make you more thirsty

- there are some artificial saliva products out there if you need them so you should ask your doctor about this

- you may need to make changes in your medications

What Are the Different Speech Therapy Techniques That Can Be Used By a Person With Parkinson's?

The following are some techniques to help with speech:

1. Pick an area that is quieter. It can be tiring to try to "talk over" the television or radio.

2. Talk slowly.

3. Be sure the person you are talking to can see your face. Look at the person while you are talking. A well-lit room can help face-to-face conversation, increasing understanding.

4. Use short phrases. Say one or two words or syllables per breath.

5. Over-articulate your speech by making your vowels longer and exaggerating the consonants.

6. Choose a comfortable posture and position that give you support during long and stressful conversations.

7. Be aware that exercises intended to strengthen weakening muscles may be counter-productive. Always ask your speech-language pathologist which exercises are right for you.

8. Plan periods of rest for your voice before you're going to have a big conversation or phone call. Know that fatigue really affects your ability to speak. Techniques that work in the morning may not work later in the day.

9. If you are soft spoken and your voice has become low, you might want to use an amplifier.

10. If you are on a respirator (with fully inflated cuffs), an electrolarynx or respiratory tube that provides an alternative air source may be used.

11. If some people have difficulty understanding you, the following ideas may help:

    - If you are able to write without too much trouble, always carry a paper and pen as a backup so you can write down what you are trying to say.

    - If writing is hard, use an alphabet board to point or scan to the first letter of the words that are spoken.

    - Spell words out loud or on an alphabet board if they are not understood.

    - Establish the topic before you speak.

    - Use telegraphic speech. Leave out words that you don't need to communicate the meaning of what you're trying to say.

    - Use expressions and gestures to communicate.

Here's a sample of the devices that are available to help people with Parkinson's disease communicate more clearly:

- **Palatal lift**. A dental apparatus that is similar to a retainer. It lifts the soft palate and stops air from escaping out of the nose during speech.

- **Amplification**. A personal amplifier can be used to increase the volume of your voice. This also decreases voice fatigue.

- **TTY telephone relay system.** A telephone that has a keyboard so speech can be typed and read by a relay operator to the listener. Either the whole message can be typed or just the words that are not understood can be typed.

- **Low technology devices**. Notebooks and language boards can be used as alternative communication techniques.

- **High technology electronic speech enhancers, communication devices.** Computers with voice synthesizers and dedicated communication devices are available.

How to communicate in an emergency:

- Use an intercom system or baby monitor to alert others that there is an emergency.

- Use bells or buzzers if you are not able to speak. Use "codes" that signify urgency. For example, ringing a bell may mean, "I'd like some company" while an air-horn means there's an emergency.

- Carry a portable phone that is has pre-programmed numbers.

- Pre-program all of your telephones so they can automatically dial the necessary emergency number(s).

- Consider a "Life Call" button if you spend time alone

Your doctor can refer you to a Speech-language pathologist who can help you. Speech-language pathologists can help people with Parkinson's disease maintain as many communication skills as possible. They also teach techniques that conserve energy, including non-verbal communication skills.

What Can Be Done to Help With Swallowing Problems?

Many people with Parkinson's disease have difficulty swallowing because they lose control of their mouth and throat muscles. Because of this, chewing and managing solid foods can be hard.

If you are having trouble swallowing, contact your doctor. He or she will recommend a speech pathologist to carefully examine your swallowing abilities and evaluate your aspiration risk.

Here are some suggestions to make chewing and swallowing easier:

- sit upright at a 90-degree angle

- tilt your head slightly forward

- remain sitting or standing up for 15-20 minutes after eating a meal

- keep the distractions to a minimum in the area where you eat

- stay focused on the tasks of eating and drinking

- don't talk with food in your mouth

- eat slowly

- cut your food into small pieces and chew it thoroughly

- don't try to eat more than 1/2 teaspoon of your food at a time

- you may need to swallow two or three times per bite or sip

- If food or liquid catches in your throat, cough gently or clear your throat, and swallow again before taking a breath. Repeat if necessary.

- concentrate on swallowing frequently

- drink plenty of fluids

- Periodically suck on popsicles, ice chips, lemon ice or lemon-flavored water to increase saliva, which will increase how often you swallow.

- Minimize (or eliminate) foods that require chewing, and eat more soft foods.

- puree your foods in a blender

- If thin liquids cause you to cough, thicken them with a liquid thickener (your speech pathologist can recommend one for you.) You can also substitute thin liquids with thicker liquid choices such as nectars for juices and cream soups for plain broths.

- When taking your medications, crush your pills and mix them with apple-sauce or pudding *Note: some pills like Sinemet CR should not be crushed because this can affect how the medications work. Ask your pharmacist for his/her recommendations on which pills shouldn't be crushed.

How Can a Person With Parkinson's Get a More Comfortable Sleep?

Here are some suggestions to help you get a more comfortable sleep.

If you have problems with moving in bed:

- try side rails, a trapeze, ropes or a handle to grip

- use satin sheets or pyjamas

- change to a firmer, lower or higher mattress

- ask a physical therapist as they may also be able to help with bed mobility, and occupational therapists may recommend other techniques

If you have foot and leg sensitivity or trouble turning in bed:

- adapt the bed with a bed hoop, blanket cradle, electric blanket or light down comforter in order to keep the bedcovers off your feet and legs

- talk to your doctor because it could be related to another medical problem

If you have problems with restless legs, painful cramping or abnormal movements:

- talk to your doctor because he or she might change the times or dosages of your medications or order other medications for pain, spasm, cramps or anxiety

- try going through some relaxation techniques or slow, relaxing stretching exercises

If you have problems with frequent urination:

- talk to your doctor or urologist to correct medical problems such as prostate problems, urinary retention or infections

- you could also put a urinal or commode near the bedside

If you are afraid of falling:

- make your home safer by getting rid of scatter rugs and putting in a nightlight

- try using a walker at night if you are able

- don't get up too quickly or you might become dizzy if you change position too quickly

If you have problems with shortness of breath, heartburn or trouble getting out of bed:

- Raise the head of the bed with blocks or extra pillows.

- Discuss shortness of breath and heartburn with your doctor.

What Can Be Done to Help a Person With PD Get More Sleep?

It is common to have problems getting enough sleep if you have PD. This may be because the part of the brain that is affected by the disease (substantia nigra) is so close to the sleep and arousal centers in the brain stem.

Medications may also sometimes be responsible. Sinemet and Parlodel can cause vivid dreams, hallucinations, leg cramps, abnormal movements and daytime drowsiness. If you don't take a diuretic early enough, you may have to get up a lot during the night to go to the bathroom.

Some tranquilizers and sleep medications commonly used stay in your system a long time and can cause daytime drowsiness that disturbs your evening's sleep.

Some breathing, seizure, high blood pressure or allergy medications can keep you up at night. Sinemet can cause this sometimes as well. Do not forget that over-the-counter pills like decongestants or antihistamines may cause sleep problems too.

Many people forget that food is often at fault. Stay away from stimulants, especially caffeine. Caffeine is found in such things as tea and chocolate as well as coffee. Alcohol may initially make you tired but can ultimately be a stimulant causing you to wake up early in the morning.

If you are having sleep problems, it is important to discuss this with your doctor and give him or her the information to help you. Think about the specifics of your problem and see if you can see a pattern. For example, if you are having painful cramping, when does it occur? When was your last dose of Sinemet before going to bed? Did the problem start after you began a new medication?

A few more tips to help you get more sleep are:

- Don't nap a lot during the day and try to have activities that keep you busy.

- Avoid using your bedroom for other activities like reading, watching TV or business.

- You can usually manage sleep problems by adjusting the timing of your medications and/or changing your diet.

- You should never take over-the-counter sleep aids without asking your doctor first. He or she can prescribe a short acting sleeping pill that doesn't interact with your PD.

- Try old time remedies like a warm glass of milk, back rubs or expressions of affection... These still work!

- Depression can often cause trouble falling asleep. Your doctor may give you an antidepressant that can also work as an anti-Parkinson's and sedative drug.

What Alternative Treatments are Available for Parkinson's?

There are several alternative therapies available for treating Parkinson's. These therapies include acupuncture, massage, yoga, tai chi, herbal and dietary therapies, (including amino acid supplementation, vitamins A, C, E, selenium and zinc therapy, B vitamin supplementation, and calcium and magnesium supplementation) as well as many others.

It's very important to note that anyone using these therapies along with conventional drugs should check with their doctor to avoid the possibility of bad interactions.

For example, vitamin B_6 (either as a supplement or from foods such as whole grains, bananas, beef, fish, liver, potatoes) can interfere with the action of L-dopa when the drug is taken without carbidopa.

The following are some alternative therapies for Parkinson's:

- **Exercise**

Although not necessarily an "alternative therapy," exercises like Tai Chi and yoga can lower your stress, help you to be more relaxed, and increase your energy, balance, and flexibility. In general, exercise is a safe, effective and easy way to improve your well-being. Remember to check with your doctor first.

- **Diet**

By following your doctor's and dietician's daily dietary guidelines, you can look and feel better with your PD. Check out the answers to **questions #83 "Is there a special diet that would help?" (p. 81)** and **#87 "What nutritional supplements help with the treatment of PD?" (p.86)** for more information about vitamin and mineral therapy.

- **Massage**

Massage can help reduce stress and tension and can loosen up tight muscles. Mom really loves this and goes once a week.

- **Acupuncture**

This is a procedure where fine needles are inserted at specific points just under the skin to stimulate, disperse and balance the flow or energy and relieve pain. You may have heard about this but have been afraid to try it. My mom certainly was but when she finally did, she couldn't believe how good it felt! She said she didn't feel the needles at all!

- **Positive Attitude**

Having a positive outlook cannot cure Parkinson's disease, but it can lower your stress and help you feel better.

- **Guided Imagery**

This is a form of focused relaxation that helps create harmony between the mind and body. Guided imagery helps you create calm, peaceful images in your mind, kind of like a "mental escape". It can help people overcome stress, anger, pain, depression, and insomnia.

Because stress and depression can worsen the symptoms of Parkinson's disease, using guided imagery can obviously be very useful to someone with PD.

First you identify your self-talk, that is, what you are saying to yourself about your life, your PD, etc. Then you make affirmations to counteract any negative thoughts and emotions.

Here are some examples of positive statements you might want to say to yourself:

- I am healthy, vital, and strong.
- Every day in every way I am getting stronger.
- There is nothing in the world I cannot handle.

- Let go of things I cannot control.

- **Homeopathy**

  Usually, the dose for the following treatments is 3 to 5 pellets of a 12X to 30C remedy every one to four hours until your symptoms get better.

- **Argentum nitricum** for ataxia (loss of muscle coordination), trembling, awkwardness, painless paralysis

- **Causticum** for Parkinson's with restless legs at night

- **Mercurius vivus** for Parkinson's that is worse at night, especially with panic attacks

- **Plumbum metallicum** especially with arteriosclerosis

- **Zincum metallicum** for great restlessness, and depression

Alternative therapy can be helpful in some cases, yet some therapies can be ineffective, costly, and even dangerous. The best way to evaluate your options is to become educated.

Weigh your options and decide whether the benefits outweigh the risks. If you do decide to try an alternative treatment, make sure your health is protected. Talk about the therapy with your doctor. Make sure your doctor knows what therapy you are considering so he or she can discuss possible interactions and/or side effects with your current treatments.

He or she can also provide you with information on other patients who may have tried the same therapy.

What is the Proper Treatment for Ongoing Acute Pain Associated With Parkinson's?

The symptoms of Parkinson's disease may cause you to move more slowly. You may also feel tightness, pain, and weakness, especially in the muscles and joints. Physical and occupational therapy may help with these symptoms.

Physical Therapy:

Physical therapy cannot cure Parkinson's disease but it can enable you to compensate for the changes in your body that you get from the disease.

A physical therapist can teach you exercises to strengthen and loosen muscles. Many of these exercises can be performed at home. The goal of physical therapy is to improve your independence and quality of life by improving movement and function and relieving pain.

Physical therapy can help with:

- Balance problems
- Lack of coordination
- Fatigue
- Pain
- Gait
- Immobility
- Weakness

Important note: Some physical therapists may apply diathermy (local heat application produced by high-frequency electrical current) to relieve muscle aches and pains. This could be dangerous to patients who have deep brain stimulators. It is very important that DBS patients inform all their health care professionals of their stimulators so potential complications can be prevented.

Occupational Therapy:

Occupational therapy can be helpful when symptoms of Parkinson's disease are making it hard for you to:

- Being productive at home or work.

- Having fun, such as enjoying pastimes and finding new ways to spend time.

- Taking care of yourself (e.g. dressing, bathing, grooming, and eating).

Occupational therapy can help people with Parkinson's disease stay active in daily life. Occupational therapists can help improve your skills, show you different ways of doing things, introduce you to handy equipment and help you perform everyday activities more easily.

An occupational therapist may also recommend making changes to your home or work to promote your independence. If you think you could benefit from occupational therapy, ask your doctor for a referral.

Here's a list of some of the areas Occupational therapists can help with:

- Arm and hand therapy
- Handwriting aids
- Information on modifying your home
- Information on driver evaluations and making modifications to your car
- Cooking and homemaking adaptations
- Eating and dinnerware adaptations
- Ways to make the most of your energy
- Computer modifications
- Workplace or work equipment modifications
- Helping you develop your leisure skills
- Manual or electric wheelchair use
- Bathtub and toilet use
- Dressing and grooming aids

For more information about pain and how to manage it, check out the **BONUS: Pain and Parkinson's Disease: Answers to Common Questions (p.119).**

How Can You Help Toe Cramping?

Here's a problem Mom has pretty frequently. She especially has this problem in the shower but it can happen anywhere.

The solution that she has found to stop the cramping is actually quite simple. She says you need to really concentrate, look down at your toes and tell them to un-cramp. It sounds simple yet it really works. Just keep looking at them and focussing and she says they will stop cramping.

What Can Be Done to Help Prevent Panic Attacks?

About 40% of people with Parkinson's are more anxious than they should be. Anxiety may be a reaction to PD or it may be part of PD, related to a loss of dopamine, norepinephrine, and serotonin nerve cells.

Researchers still haven't figured out for sure what factors cause anxiety in people with Parkinson's.

Some studies have shown that Levodopa therapy could possibly cause panic attacks.

Panic attacks are outbursts of anxiety that can be triggered by many things. These attacks can last for periods of time between a few seconds and a few hours.

If you are having a panic attack, you may feel things like shortness of breath, clammy sweat, irregular heartbeat, dizziness, faintness, and feelings of unreality.

A panic attack may be triggered by many things such as a fear of dying, fear of going insane, breathlessness, sweating, chest discomfort, choking, and dizziness.

A panic attack can sometimes look like a heart attack, and, sometimes, you will have to make sure that it's not a heart attack. In many people the panic attacks happen only in certain situations and may be linked to immobility.

For instance, in people who have "on/off" episodes, panic attacks almost always occur during the "off" period. When panic attacks occur during the "off" period, their intensity parallels the difference in mobility between the "off" and the "on."

In these people treatment should be directed toward decreasing the fluctuations.

In some people, panic attacks may happen throughout the day, regardless of whether they are "on" or "off." Serotonin re-uptake inhibitors, a type of antidepressant, are also useful in treating panic attacks.

A lot of times, anxiety is seen together with depression. Studies have shown that possibly as much as 92% of Parkinson's people who have had an anxiety disorder have also had a depressive disorder.

It would make sense then, that treating the depression could play an important part in treating the anxiety.

There are quite a lot of available treatments for people who suffer anxiety. Unfortunately, very little research has been done to figure out the best course of treatment for those who have panic attacks.

Here's a list of some drugs that are available for treatment of anxiety: (Yikes! Some of these drug names are pretty long. Your doctor will know more about them. Ask him or her about which drugs would be best for you)

- Tricyclic Antidepressants

- Selective serotonin reuptake inhibitors

- Nonselective monoamine oxidase inhibitors (Risk of hypertension when taken with levodopa)

- Benzodiazepines (Can worsen Parkinsonian symptoms when taking high dosages)

- Busiprone

Is There An Operation for People With PD Which Can Improve Their Quality of Life?

There are a few operations that can help improve the quality of life in someone with Parkinson's. Not all operations are for everybody, and it's best to read up on them and discuss them with your doctor to find out if you might be a good candidate for any one of them.

1a. Deep Brain Stimulation (DBS):

Deep brain stimulation is a way to inactivate the parts of the brain that cause Parkinson's, without purposefully destroying the brain.

In deep brain stimulation, electrodes are placed in the part of the brain called the globus pallidus. The electrodes are connected by wires to a type of pacemaker device (called an impulse generator, or IPG) implanted under the skin of the chest, below the collarbone.

Once it's activated, the device sends continuous electrical pulses to the target areas in the brain, blocking the impulses that cause tremors.

This has the same effect as thalamotomy or pallidotomy surgeries without actually destroying parts of the brain.

The IPG can easily be programmed using a computer that sends radio signals to the device. Patients are given special magnets so they can externally turn the IPG on or off.

Depending on use, the stimulators may last three to five years. Replacing the IPG is a pretty simple procedure as well.

DBS has been successful in treating people of different ages. However, each person has to be assessed individually to see if they have the stamina and overall health before considering surgery.

Surgery is not recommended if the medications you are taking are still helping the symptoms of your PD. However, surgery should be considered for people who do not achieve satisfactory control with medications. Talk to your doctor to see if DBS is right for you.

1b. Subthalamic Nucleus Deep Brain Stimulation:

Subthalamic Nucleus Stimulation is a new form of the original DBS technique.

Subthalamic nucleus DBS has been recognized as the most effective surgical treatment for Parkinson's disease because it treats not only the tremors, but also the rigidity, slowness of movement, stiffness, and problems with walking and balance.

People who have this surgery often experience a great reduction in their dyskinesia mostly because they are able to reduce their medications following the surgery.

In addition to this, the surgery to place the stimulator in the subthalamic nucleus is generally easier than surgeries for the thalamus or globus pallidus.

Advantages of Deep Brain Stimulation:

- First, it does not require purposeful destruction of any part of the brain and therefore, has fewer complications than thalamotomy and pallidotomy.

- In addition, the electrical stimulation is adjustable and can be changed as the person's disease changes or his or her response to medications change. No further surgery is necessary to make the adjustments.

- Another significant advantage of deep brain stimulation relates to future treatments. Destructive surgery, like thalamotomy or pallidotomy, may reduce the persons' potential to benefit from future therapies.

For example, future brain cell transplantation may be of great help to people with Parkinson's disease. There is concern that a pallidotomy or thalamotomy may prevent patients from benefiting from brain cell transplantation. This would not be the case with deep brain stimulation, as the stimulator could be turned off.

- Deep brain stimulation is a relatively safe procedure.

- The procedure can treat all the major symptoms of Parkinson's disease.

- Daily living tasks and quality of life are also improved.

- With subthalamic nucleus stimulation, medications can usually be reduced.

- The stimulator can also be turned off at any time if deep brain stimulation is causing excessive side effects.

- The vast majority of people (over 70%) experience a significant improvement of all their symptoms related to Parkinson's disease. Most people are able to significantly reduce their medications.

- Most people experience little discomfort during the procedure.

Possible Disadvantages of Deep Brain Stimulation:

- Increased risk of infection. Implanting any foreign object in your body carries that risk.

- Additional surgery may be needed if the equipment stops working or for battery replacement.

- It will take time to adjust your medications afterwards.

- As with any surgical procedure, there are risks. There is a 2%-3% risk of a serious and permanent complication such as paralysis, changes in thinking, memory and personality, seizures, and infection. Talk to your doctor to see if these risks apply to you.

- DBS of the globus pallidus seems to be somewhat less effective for problems with walking and balance than does Subthalamic DBS.

- Some devices, like theft detectors and screening devices (like those found in airports, department stores and public libraries) can cause your neurotransmitter to switch on or off.

Usually, this only causes an uncomfortable sensation. However, your symptoms could get worse suddenly. Always carry the identification card given to you. With this, you may request assistance to bypass those devices.

2. Pallidotomy:

It is thought that the part of the brain called the globus pallidus becomes overactive in Parkinson's disease. This over activity acts like a brake and slows or diminishes bodily movement.

Pallidotomy surgery permanently destroys the overactive globus pallidus to lessen the symptoms of Parkinson's disease. This treatment can eliminate rigidity and significantly reduce tremor, bradykinesia, and balance problems.

Pallidotomy can also help the medications work better in people with an advanced form of Parkinson's disease.

3. Thalamotomy:

It is thought that the abnormal brain activity that causes tremor is processed through the thalamus. Thalamotomy destroys part of the thalamus to block the abnormal brain activity from reaching the muscles and causing tremor.

Because thalamotomy is used only to control tremors, it is not generally recommended as a treatment for Parkinson's disease.

Although thalamotomy and pallidotomy surgeries are still done today, they are done less frequently because of the risk of serious side effects and the availability of deep brain stimulation, which is safer and has fewer complications.

4. Gamma Knife:

The gamma knife is a machine that shoots out hundreds of powerful, highly focused gamma radiation beams. The gamma knife allows for a more precise and concentrated treatment than do other radiation treatment options.

This helps the doctors target the diseased area of the brain while sparing the healthy areas surrounding it.

Even though it is not as effective as deep brain stimulation, gamma knife does offer another treatment option for some who may not be able to undergo deep brain stimulation surgery.

For example, some people taking anti-coagulant medicines (blood-thinners) can't go without their medicine even for a short period of time. For these people, a non-invasive surgical approach, like gamma knife surgery, may be beneficial.

Gamma knife treatment is considered only when a person is not able to get relief from medication and when deep brain stimulation, which is a more effective therapy, is not appropriate.

There are many important issues to be addressed when considering gamma knife treatment. You should talk to your doctor about these before considering this surgery.

Patients who undergo the gamma knife treatment experience very little, if any, discomfort and serious side effects are rare. Gamma knife treatment usually is performed on an outpatient basis.

The benefits of gamma knife treatment occur over time, usually several months to several years, depending on the person's medical condition.

Gamma knife treatment has up to a 70%-90% success rate, which depends on the patient.

As with all surgical procedures, there is a small risk of complications. Make sure you talk to your doctor about these risks when considering gamma knife treatment.

Gamma knife treatment is not considered experimental. Many insurance carriers provide coverage for this procedure.

Are There Any Developments Leading to Better Treatment for Parkinson's?

Because researchers' understanding of how the brain works has greatly increased in recent years, many believe that a cure for Parkinson's may be just around the corner.

There is research being done on something called embryonic stem cells. This is pretty controversial research and involves stem cells from embryos that are a few days old. Most of these embryos result from in vitro fertilization efforts.

Stem cells are the parent cells of all tissues in the body. This means they can turn in to any type of cell. The hope is that they will eventually be able to make these cells into specific types of cells, like dopamine-producing neurons, that can be used to treat Parkinson's disease.

There is also hope that adult stem cells, which are harvested from bone marrow, might be able to work the same way as embryonic stem cells.

There are fewer ethical questions about this kind of research, but some researchers believe that adult stem cells may be more difficult to work with than those from embryos.

Either way, most all researchers believe that working on all forms of stem cells is important for the continuation of their work.

Some researchers are looking at the possible role of genetic and environmental factors in causing Parkinson's. Making progress in discovering what causes Parkinson's will open a whole new world of research into curing the disease.

In the end, the more research that can be done, the sooner a cure or new therapies that can stop the progression of the disease will be discovered.

What Is Fetal Cell Transplantation?

Fetal cell transplantation is a procedure in which fetal cells are implanted into the brains of people with Parkinson's disease to replace the dopamine-producing cells in the substantia nigra.

Although promising, this area of research is one of the most controversial. Some studies have found that fetal cell transplantation caused an increase in severe involuntary movements (dyskinesia) due to too much dopamine in the brain. There are also moral and ethical objections to the use of fetal cell implants. As a result, other methods of treatment are being explored.

Some of these methods include the use of cells from other mammals, cells from human placentas or umbilical cords, and synthetic microspheres (basically really small sponge-like balls) that deliver dopamine directly to the brain.

Some researchers hope to use cloning techniques on animal fetuses as a source for dopamine-producing nerve cells. Animal and laboratory studies are also using gene therapies and other advanced treatments for transplanting dopamine-producing cells or nerve-protecting cells into the brain.

How Can Stem Cells Help Someone With Parkinson's?

Stem cells are the parent cells of all tissues in the body. This means they can turn in to any type of cell. The hope is that they will eventually be able to make these cells into specific types of cells, like dopamine-producing neurons, that can be used to treat Parkinson's disease.

However, there are concerns that patients may have the same risk of increased involuntary movements as those who undergo fetal cell transplantation. And, like fetal cell transplantation, stem cell therapy is surrounded by moral and ethical controversy.

Where Can I Find More Information About the Most Recent Parkinson's Treatments?

There are definitely many resources out there for information but your best bet is to start with your National Parkinson's Foundation. They can put you in touch with many resources and can provide books, pamphlets and videos regarding the types of treatment available.

One resource Mom has found to be very handy is a Parkinson's magazine which she subscribed to through her National PD Foundation and this has very up to date information on the new medications, surgeries, and the current research that is being done.

You can also try looking in your local phone book in the yellow and/or white pages for your local Parkinson's chapter, as well as the library.

Most of all National Foundations also have websites where you can get more information and contact numbers if you need them.

How Can People With Parkinson's Make Their Life Better?

To start off, you must not be afraid to ask for help when you think you need it. Yes, it's important to keep your independence as long as possible, but this doesn't mean that you can't have a little help along the way.

A few things Mom said were important for her were first to think long term. Ask yourself "How's this going to work for me down the road?" when thinking about making changes to your house, or even buying new clothing. It's not meant to be depressing, just practical.

Always allow extra time for everything so you won't be rushed. Every time Mom starts to feel rushed, she just about shuts down and then we can't go anywhere.

Also, if getting ready to go out takes up all your energy so that you end up not enjoying your outing, you need to get help in getting ready. Don't try to be too independent, Mom says.

Another thing Mom says is very important is to concentrate on one task at a time. People with PD often tend to jump from one task to another without completing either of them so concentrating could help you get more things done.

Getting discouraged while exercising is something that happens even to the best of us. Try not to get discouraged if your exercise is difficult. Keep trying and don't give up!

Finally, support groups can be very helpful, especially if you have problems talking to your doctor. Connecting with other people who really know what it is like to have Parkinson's disease can be very helpful in coping.

Support groups offer a safe place to talk about your feelings, questions and concerns and to get valuable information. There are many available Parkinson's support groups in the community that are free of charge. Most cities have some form of a support group, and if not, a list of support groups will be available with your National Parkinson's foundation.

Here are some more things you can do to make your life better:

- **Be Informed**

Learn as much as you can about Parkinson's and its treatment (like reading this book!) Knowledge is power. The more you understand, the more you can discuss with your doctor about your treatment.

- **Socialize**

Isolation can only make you feel worse if you are depressed. It is important to keep up your social life, be involved in activities that you like and talk things over with your family and friends. Dealing with Parkinson's is not something you need to do by yourself. Your family and friends will want to be involved in helping you.

- **Do Things You Enjoy**

Doing something fun that gets your mind off of Parkinson's disease can be really helpful in coping with the disease. Go to a movie, listen to some beautiful music, read a good book, garden or help other people.

- **Don't Be Afraid!**

Don't be afraid to ask your doctor to repeat any instructions or medical terms that you don't understand or remember. It's very important that you are able to talk things over with your doctor and not be afraid of what he or she might say. Doctors should always be available to answer your questions and address your concerns.

- **Learn to Manage Stress**

This will help you to maintain a positive physical, emotional, and spiritual outlook on life. Being stressed out will only make the situation worse. You should try to organize a daily routine that will reduce stress, with down time for both you and your family members.

- **Exercise**

Exercise has been found to be very helpful in minimizing the symptoms of Parkinson's disease, increasing mobility and improving quality of life. It can also be very emotionally beneficial. It has been found to help in improve a depressed or anxious mood. Consider trying yoga or Tai Chi, which are relaxing and improve flexibility and balance.

- **Counselling**

You may find it helpful to find a counsellor for yourself and/or your family. Counsellors can be very helpful in dealing with the emotional issues you might be facing with Parkinson's. If you decide this is for you, your doctor can provide you with a referral. Your doctor might also prescribe antidepressants if you are depressed.

- **Positive/Hopeful Attitude**

Yes, the disease may be out of your control, but you do have control over your attitude towards it. It is important not to let the disease define who you are. Focus on all the other aspects of your life that are positive. Be thankful for all that you have. Don't beat yourself up about things because it will only make things worse.

- **Humor**

There is definitely some truth to the adage, "Laughter is the best medicine". Being able to laugh a little about your situation helps to keep it in perspective and relieves some of the stress. It can also help in awkward situations because it tends to put people around you at ease, and that often opens up communication.

- **Take Care of Yourself**

Treating Parkinson's involves more than just medications. Diet, exercise, support from friends and family, as well as a good attitude all need to be a part of your treatment. Be good to yourself, be patient with yourself and be a friend to yourself. You deserve it!

NUTRITION AND EXERCISE

Is There a Special Diet That Would Help?

Although there is no special diet required for people with Parkinson's disease, eating a well-balanced, nutritious diet is really helpful. With the proper diet, your body works more efficiently, has more energy, and your medications will work properly.

As always, it is important to talk to your doctor and possibly a nutritionist before you make any changes in your diet.

As a general rule, you should eat a variety of foods from each food category, and ask your doctor if you should take a daily vitamin supplement.

Here's a list of some other foods you may want to add to your diet that may help your PD:

Foods To Eat:

- **Water!**

   Drink at least six to eight 8-ounce glasses of pure water daily to help flush toxins from your body.

- **Glutamine**

   Raising glutamine levels (a potent antioxidant and detoxifier) will provide a protective effect.

- **Amino acids**

   Low-protein diets may help control tremors. However, D-tyrosine (100 mg per kg per day) increases dopamine turnover.

- **Raw seeds** (such as sunflower and pumpkin)

- **Sprouted grains**

- **Seaweeds**

- **Vegetable juice** (especially carrot)

- **Vegetables** (especially leafy greens)

- **Fruit**

    Fruits are a good source of antioxidants.

- **Fibre**

    People often eat bran in hopes of helping relieve constipation that results from their PD.

    Recent research shows that bran is high in vitamin B-6, which interferes with the effectiveness of levodopa when the drug is taken alone.

    Instead of bran, try prune juice, grains, and fibre laxatives. You may also want to include high-fibre foods such as vegetables, cooked dried peas and beans (legumes), whole-grain foods, cereals, pasta, rice, and fresh fruit in your diet.

- **Spelt** (made as congee)

    Spelt is an ancient grain that is a nutritious and flavorful relative of wheat. It has been used in the treatment of many disorders, including Parkinson's.

- **Fava beans**

    Also called broad beans, are a natural source of levodopa. One-half cup contains 250 mg, or the same amount as one pill. But don't substitute beans for pills without first asking your doctor.

- **Grape Seed Extract** (Pycnogenol)

    Flavonoids, and in particular the proanthocyanidins (grape seed and pine bark extracts) have been found to help prevent and slow the progression of PD.

    Proanthocyanidins are water-soluble antioxidants that are stronger than vitamin C and which can quickly cross into the brain fluid.

- **Caffeine/Coffee**

    A team of researchers looked at the relationship between coffee intake and the incidence of Parkinson's disease among 8,004 Japanese-American men over a 30 year period.

Of these men, 102 developed Parkinson's disease. People who drank coffee were less likely to get PD. In fact, the men who drank the most coffee were the least likely to get Parkinson's disease.

Men who did not drink any coffee were five times more likely to show symptoms of Parkinson's disease than men who drank more than 28 ounces of coffee each day.

Caffeine from other sources such as green tea, black tea, chocolate and soda were also associated with a lower risk of Parkinson's disease.

It is thought that caffeine may protect against Parkinson's disease by blocking something called adenosine receptors, and increasing the amount of dopamine in the brain.

Though there may be a link between caffeine and PD, it is too early to say that caffeine will prevent Parkinson's disease. Maybe the brains of people who like and dislike coffee are different, with differing rates of Parkinson's.

The study also included older, Japanese-American men which means we don't know if this caffeine/Parkinson disease relationship would be the same for other ethnic groups, women or younger people.

How Much Protein is Allowed in a Parkinson's Diet?

First of all, a person with PD needs to consider how severe their symptoms are. If a person has problems with mobility that interfere with activities or has noticed that food seems to interfere with how well Sinemet works, a low protein diet may help these problems.

People who need to lower the protein in their diet might try reducing it to the recommended daily allowance of protein. The recommended daily allowance (RDA) for protein is .8 grams of protein per kilogram of body weight (.36 grams per pound).

Timing when you eat protein is important as well. If you have most of your protein at your evening meal, you will increase the amount of time you are mobile. But, if you evenly distribute your protein throughout the day, you will be less mobile in the evenings.

You will have to decide which option is best for you and your needs, but in the meantime, here are a few ways to incorporate protein into your mealtimes so that it won't interfere with the effectiveness of Sinemet:

- Take Sinemet about 30 minutes before meals

- Eat foods that are high in protein, with large helpings of grains, fruits, and vegetables

- Remember that meals high in fat take longer to digest

Remember if you do cut down on your protein, you may want take vitamin and mineral supplements as a low-protein diet can lead to low levels of calcium, iron, and B vitamins.

Are There Certain Foods That People With Parkinson's Should Avoid?

The following are some suggestions on foods that a person with Parkinson's might avoid.

Foods to avoid if you have Parkinson's:

- **Tobacco**

- **Spicy Foods**

Foods seasoned with hot spices have been known to cause uncontrollable physical movement in some people with Parkinson's.

- **Aspartame** (NutraSweet)

Parkinson's disease can be triggered or worsened by ingesting aspartame according to researchers studying its possible adverse effects.

- **High Protein**

High amounts of protein in the diet decrease the effectiveness of Sinemet. The timing of protein intake can increase the effectiveness of Sinemet and make it so you don't require as much medication.

- **Alcohol**

This creates an acidic internal environment and is over- stimulating to a stressed nervous system.

Foods, minerals and metals to avoid that help decrease risk of Parkinson's:

- **Chemicalized and Processed Food**

As much as possible, buy organic fruits, vegetables, and grains to lower the amount of **exposure you get to pesticide residues**. (Direct contact with herbicides and pesticides can put you at increased risk of Parkinson's)

- **Animal/ Saturated Fats**

American researchers have concluded that a high intake of animal fats is associated with a **five-fold increase in the risk** of developing Parkinson's disease

- **Sugar**

People with a high intake of sugar (mono- and disaccharides) may increase their risk of developing Parkinson's disease by a factor of three as compared to people with a more moderate intake.

Minerals:

- **Iron**

Avoiding overexposure to some metals, especially iron, may help reduce the risk of developing Parkinson's disease.

- **Manganese**

- **Copper**

Metals:

- **Aluminum**

People who live in areas where the aluminum content of the drinking water is high might have a higher risk of developing Parkinson's disease.

Are There Any Food Additives That a Person With Parkinson's Should Avoid?

There have been studies that have suggested that something called "excitatory amino acids" might play a role in Parkinson's disease.

These types of amino acids are found naturally in many protein food sources and are often added to food in the form of monosodium glutamate (MSG), a flavor enhancer you've probably heard about (if you haven't, check out the labels of your soup cans-it's often in the ingredients list).

The studies that have been done haven't been conclusive yet but some researchers have said it might be a good idea to limit the use of MSG and similar additives, as well as the artificial sweetener aspartame. ***NOTE:** For more information on MSG and how it may be harmful to you, checkout the articles about MSG at the end of the **bonus book "Making Life With Parkinson's Easier".** You can find the articles on pages 260-266 .

What Nutritional Supplements Help With the Treatment of Parkinson's?

Well, there's a lot of information out there about taking this, that or the other thing to help with your Parkinson's. Some say one thing works, and others say it doesn't. Obviously, you need to talk to your doctor about this but here are some recommendations that some researchers have found to help with PD.

Vitamins and Minerals:

- **Multivitamin**

These are great to help out your diet if you aren't getting all the vitamins and minerals you need. Try taking a high-potency multivitamin and mineral supplement daily. Soft gel-caps are the best form of multivitamin because you can digest them easier.

- **Vitamin B6**

Vitamin B6 is recommended regardless of the cause of the disease and of the patient's age, and can be given either alone or in combination with anti-Parkinsonian drugs aside from DOPA. (10 to 100 mg per day may help with symptom control, but should be given with 30 mg per day of zinc).

High doses of B6 are not recommended, however, for people with angina or coronary insufficiency.

NOTE: Vitamin B6 (also called pyridoxine), found in bananas, beef, fish, liver, oatmeal, peanuts, potatoes, and whole grains, interferes with the action of L-dopa. If you are taking L-dopa, take these foods only in moderation, if at all. (If you are taking a combination Levadopa and cardidopa such as Sinemet, you don't have to avoid the intake of Vitamin B6.)

- **Vitamin E**

A study showed that taking large amounts of vitamin E (from food only) reduced the risk of Parkinson's disease. This study involved over 124 000 men and women who were followed for at least 12 years.

Vitamin E supplements were NOT associated with the risk of developing Parkinson's (taking 400 to 800 IU per day).

NOTE: If you have high blood pressure, limit your intake of supplemental vitamin E to a total of 400 international units daily. If you are taking an anticoagulant (blood thinner), consult your physician before taking supplemental vitamin E.

- **Vitamin C**

Some studies have shown that supplementing your diet with vitamin C can really slow down the progression of the disease in its early stages and may be an excellent protector against Parkinson's disease (taking 1,000 mg three times a day).

Other research has shown that synthetic vitamin E (this is vitamin E that is still in the pill form, but just has "synthetic" as opposed to "natural" written on the side of the bottle) by itself may not slow the progression of Parkinson's disease, but in combination with vitamin C, it may.

- **Vitamin A**

Vitamin A works with other antioxidants (like vitamin E and C) to provide a protective effect.

- **Vitamin B Complex**

Adding a vitamin B-complex to your diet may be necessary, especially if you take L-dopa medications.

- **Trace Mineral Selenium**

Taking 200 mcg may slow down the progression of Parkinson's. Selenium is an antioxidant that works with vitamin E. It also helps to increase circulation and tissue oxygenation, thereby limiting damage to nerve cells.

- **Calcium and Magnesium**

These are very important for maintaining a healthy nervous system. Take a multimineral supplement that supplies 500 milligrams of calcium and 250 milligrams of magnesium, as well as trace minerals, twice daily.

- **Folic Acid**

Folic acid is a B vitamin. It is used in our bodies to make new cells.

Some studies have shown that low levels of folic acid increase your chances of getting Parkinson's disease.

Researchers think that consuming enough amounts of folate or folic acid may help protect older adults from Parkinson's disease as well as from other degenerative neurological diseases.

Folate naturally occurs in dark green vegetables like spinach, in citrus fruits, and in whole-wheat bread. Half a cup of cooked spinach contains about 130 micrograms of folate.

Nutrients:

- **CoQ10** (Ubiquinone)

Researchers have done a study where they found that Parkinson's patients have reduced levels of coenzyme Q10 in their mitochondria (cells' power sources).

This led the researchers to see whether the antioxidant would be useful in treating the disease.

In their study there were 80 people who had been diagnosed with Parkinson's who had not received treatment yet. These people were randomly assigned to take a daily dose of 300mg, 600mg or 1,200mg of coenzyme Q10 or an inactive pill called a placebo. They were evaluated at the start of the study and after one, four, eight, twelve and sixteen months.

The progression of Parkinson's disease was a lot slower in people taking the highest dose of coenzyme Q10. These people experienced a slower decline in all the areas measured by the researchers, including mental and motor skills, but the greatest effect was in the activities of daily living.

The results of this study suggest that doses of coenzyme Q_{10} as high as 1,200 mg/day are safe (30 milligrams two or three times daily is the average dose) and may be more effective than lower doses.

- **Alpha Lipoic Acid**

Alpha-lipoic acid is an antioxidant that also helps to "recharge" other antioxidants in the body. Take 50 to 100 milligrams three times a day.

- **TMG (Tri-methyl-glycine)/SAMe**

TMG is a nutrient that can enable a person to function at more optimum mental and physical levels. It helps the body in overcoming a number of bad health conditions, and is an important part of human metabolism. TMG has been shown to improve Parkinson's disease.

- **Essential Fatty Acids**

These are anti-inflammatory. A mix of omega-6 (evening primrose, black currant, borage, pumpkin seed) and omega-3 (flaxseed and fish oils) may be best (2 tbsp. oil per day or 1,000 to 1,500 mg twice a day).

Herbs:

Herbs may be used as dried extracts (capsules, powders, teas), glycerites (glycerine extracts), or tinctures (alcohol extracts). Unless otherwise indicated, teas should be made with 1 tsp. herb per cup of hot water. Steep, covered 5 to 10 minutes for leaf or flowers, and 10 to 20 minutes for roots. Drink 2 to 4 cups per day.

- **Gotu kola** (Centella asiatica):

This herb was used historically to treat Parkinson's disease.

Gotu kola has been known to have remarkable wound healing properties, as well as improving memory and increasing mental stamina. Dosage is one cup tea twice a day, or 30 to 60 drops tincture twice a day.

- **Ginkgo** (Ginkgo biloba):

Taken as a supplement of 120 mg per day, Ginkgo biloba chases after and captures free radicals, as well as boosts circulation to the brain. It has been found to be especially helpful in cases dementia and Alzheimer's disease. Mom says she finds it helps her remember things better.

Select a product containing at least 24 percent ginkgo heterosides (sometimes called flavoglycosides). If you feel fine with the 120 mg dosage, you can gradually increase to as much as 80 milligrams three times daily.

- **Hawthorn** (Crataegus monogyna):

  Taking 2 to 5 g per day, it increases the efficiency of the heart by increasing circulation, it helps to stop palpitations and arrhythmias, and helps to prevent and treat angina.

- **Milk thistle** (Silybum marianum), globe artichoke (Cynara scolymus), and Bupleurum species:

  Provide support for the liver.

- **St. John's wort** (Hypericum perforatum), skullcap (Scutellaria lateriflora), oats (Avena sativa), and lemon balm (Melissa officinalis):

  Help support the structure of the nervous system.

Does Exercise Help Parkinson's?

Because Parkinson's disease affects your ability to move, exercise helps to keep muscles strong and improve flexibility and mobility. Exercise will not stop the disease from progressing but it will improve your balance and it can prevent joint stiffening.

Exercise has been found to be very helpful in minimizing the symptoms of Parkinson's disease, increasing mobility and improving quality of life. It can also be very emotionally beneficial. It has been found to help in improving a depressed or anxious mood.

You should check with your doctor before beginning any exercise program. Your doctor may make recommendations about:

- The types of exercise best suited to you, and those which you should avoid

- The intensity of the workout (how hard you should be working)

- The duration of your workout and any physical limitations

- Referrals to other professionals, such as a physical therapist who can help you create your own personal exercise program

Are There Any Special Exercise Regimens That Are Recommended for a Person With PD?

The type of exercise that works best for you depends on your symptoms, fitness level, and overall health. Generally, exercises that stretch your arms and legs through the full range of motion are encouraged.

It's important that you find a kind of exercise that you enjoy, or else you're probably not going to stick with it. Mom likes puttering around in her garden and going for walks when she's mobile (she also has a treadmill that she can use inside when the weather's not so great).

Some other ideas other than gardening and walking are; swimming, water aerobics (easier on the joints and require less balance), yoga and Tai Chi (both of which are relaxing and improve flexibility and balance).

Here are some tips to keep in mind when exercising:

- Talk to your doctor first about what exercise you think you might like to do and whether or not it's a good choice for your overall health.

- Always warm-up before beginning your exercise routine and cool down at the end.

- If you plan to workout for 30 minutes, start with 10-minute sessions and work your way up.

- Exercise the muscles in your face, jaw, and voice when possible: Sing or read aloud, exaggerating your lip movements. Make faces in the mirror. Chew food vigorously.

- Work out in a safe place; avoid slippery floors, poor lighting, throw rugs, and other possible hazards.

- If you have difficulty balancing, exercise within reach of a grab bar or rail. If you have trouble standing or getting up, try exercising in bed rather than on the floor or an exercise mat.

- If at any time you feel sick or you begin to hurt, stop.

- Pick an exercise, activity or hobby you enjoy and stick with it.

What is Tai Chi and Can it Help Someone With Parkinson's?

Tai chi is a martial art developed in fourteenth century China. In the tradition of karate and judo, tai chi was originally used for self-defence, and has evolved over the course of time into a practice for promoting health.

Tai Chi is also a philosophy. It's the philosophy of yin and yang. Literally, it means "supreme ultimate." Tai chi is represented by the yin/yang symbol. It's sort of the law of opposites (like you and me, night and day, etc.). Through the movements, you're trying to bring your body, mind and nature together to become one.

You've probably seen someone in a park sometime doing a very beautiful, slow, ballet-like series of motions that looked a little strange to you if you didn't know what it was, because there are many people now practicing this on their own. If you saw someone doing that in the park in your town, it was probably tai chi.

Tai Chi has been recommended for helping people with Parkinson's because it is relaxing and can improve flexibility and balance. Whether you take a class or practice on your own, you may want to try this exercise as part of your PD treatment plan.

Is Weight Loss a Symptom of Parkinson's or a Side Effect of the Drugs?

Many people with PD lose weight because of the nausea, stress, and loss of appetite that they get from the disease and the drugs.

Losing weight may weaken your immune system, cause you to lose muscle and you may also be missing out on important nutrients.

Because of this, it's really important to eat healthy, well-balanced meals. If you find that you can't eat a lot at once, eat 5-6 smaller meals over the course of the day. You may also try a meal supplement such as Ensure.

How Can a Person With Parkinson's Maintain Body Weight?

Here are some general tips to help you maintain a healthy weight:

- Weigh yourself once or twice a week, unless your doctor recommends weighing yourself more often. If you are taking diuretics or steroids, such as prednisone, you should weigh yourself daily.

- If you have an unexplained weight gain or loss (2 pounds in one day or 5 pounds in one week), talk to your doctor. He or she may want to change your food or fluid intake to help manage your condition.

Here are some tips for gaining weight:

- Ask your doctor about nutritional supplements. Sometimes supplements in the form of snacks, drinks (such as Ensure or Boost), or vitamins may be prescribed to eat between meals to help you increase your calories and get the right amount of nutrients every day.

  Make sure you check with your doctor before making any dietary changes or before adding supplements to your diet. Some can be harmful or interfere with your medication.

- Avoid low-fat or low-calorie products (unless your doctor has recommended otherwise). Use whole milk, whole milk cheese, and yogurt.

Sometimes you might be losing weight because you don't have much of an appetite.

Here are some tips for improving poor appetite:

- Talk to your doctor; sometimes, poor appetite is due to depression, which can be treated. Your appetite will probably improve after depression is treated.

- Avoid non-nutritious drinks like black coffee and tea.

- Eat small, frequent meals and snacks.

- Walk or get involved in another light activity to stimulate your appetite.

Here are some tips to help you eat more at meals:

- Have your drinks after a meal instead of before or during a meal so that you do not feel full before you start eating.

- Plan meals to include your favorite foods.

- Try eating the high-calorie foods in your meal first.

- Increase the variety of food you're eating (use your imagination, or a good cookbook)

Here are some tips to help you eat snacks:

- Don't waste your energy eating foods that have little or no nutritional value like potato chips, candy bars, colas and other snack foods.

- Choose high-protein and high-calorie snacks. Some examples of these kind of snacks are: ice cream, cookies, pudding, cheese, granola bars, custard, sandwiches, nachos with cheese, eggs, crackers with peanut butter, bagels with peanut butter or cream cheese, cereal with half and half, fruit or vegetables with dips, yogurt with granola, popcorn with margarine and parmesan cheese, bread sticks with cheese sauce.

- Make food preparation easy. Choose foods that are easy to make and eat.

- Make eating a good experience, not a chore. To liven things up at meal times, try putting on background music and using colorful place settings.

- Try not to eat alone. Invite somebody over for dinner or go out.

CAREGIVING

What Can You Do to Help Someone You Know With Parkinson's Realize They Need Help?

Let's assume that you know someone with Parkinson's who is living on their own and has so far refused help from anyone, despite the fact that they probably need it.

First off, if they have refused treatment altogether (including medications), you might tell them that research has shown that you may be able to slow down the progression of the disease if you start treatment sooner than later.

If they are taking medications for their PD but are still requiring some help with their daily activities, you may suggest a home support worker, or someone who could help them out from time to time (like a family member or friend).

This might be a good option for them, especially if they are afraid of losing their independence. The support worker (or whoever) could come out on a trial basis and that way the person could see what the benefits of having outside help are.

Express to them your concerns about them refusing help. Would they be able to help themselves in an emergency? They need to know that in the end, help is there to make them feel better, not worse.

What Are Some Practical Ways a Caregiver Can Make Life Easier for Someone With Parkinson's as the Disease Progresses?

Caregivers can help in many ways to help make the life of a person with Parkinson's easier. To start, Mom says it's very good to be supportive, encouraging, and positive.

Try to avoid stressful situations if at all possible. Try to talk in a "happy voice" Mom says, because the Parkinsonian can hear (yes, not just see, but hear as well!) when you are stressed and this stress really affects them negatively.

Because depression is so common, it never hurts to offer a hug or two, or any kind of physical touch. Mom really appreciates these I know.

As much as possible, be accessible. Ask if you can help them, but don't assume they want help because they may not. Asking is important because often the person with Parkinson's won't ask for help for fear they are being a pain all the time.

You may want to participate in their exercise program with them if they have one, to help them stay motivated.

One very important thing you need to know as a caregiver for someone with Parkinson's is that patience goes a long way. You need to remember that things will often take longer than they might have before and trying to rush someone with PD will only get them frustrated and stressed and slow them down even more.

Always PLAN AHEAD and allow extra time for things. Mom loves to shop and some days we can get ready in 15 minutes to go to the mall, while other times it may take an hour. "It's okay" we tell her," 'cause the mall ain't goin' nowhere!"

How Can I Take Advantage of Outside Help Without My Loved-One (who has PD) Getting Upset?

First of all, you need to help make your loved one understand why you need help. You might explain about burnout and how this will eventually happen to you if you don't get outside help. This will mean that you will no longer be able to care for them.

Next, you need to explain why having some outside help in the home could be good. Mention to them that this could be a way to learn new things, as well as having some new company in the house for him or her. You might suggest having a "trial" period so that the both of you could see how and if this would be good for your situation.

Finally, remind them that in the end, what helps you as the caregiver will also help them.

What Resources are Available for Caregivers?

There are many resources available for caregivers, but the best place to start is with your National Parkinson's Foundation or Society. They can quickly and easily direct you to the best places for you to get the resources you want and need. You can find them online, or in the phone book.

The next place you might try looking is in your local newspaper for community announcements of meetings for caregivers. You can also try looking in the yellow and/or white pages of your phone book for your local Parkinson's chapter, who will be able to tell you about any support groups that may be in your area.

MISCELLANEOUS

Are There Any Organizations That Give Monetary Support for a Person With Parkinson's?

Outside of government funding, there aren't a whole lot of organizations that give straight cash. Well, not that we could find anyway (If you know of some, let us know!).

One non-government organization that we found that does help is called "The Melvin Weinstein Parkinson's Foundation". This a non-profit organization dedicated to purchasing equipment and health supplies necessary to maintain a safe and healthy environment for Parkinson's Patients. With the aid of support groups they locate Parkinson's Patients who have financial and medical needs, and find a way to help them.

The best way to receive monetary support is through either employment disability benefits, or various federal health and or disability support plans.

Do People With Parkinson's Receive Any Financial Help From the Government?

Yes! It is possible that you may qualify to receive financial help from your government. It is very important that you investigate this to see if you qualify because there are many ways in which they might be able to help you.

First of all, your condition will need to be assessed to see what stage of the disease you're in and what assistive devices (if any) would make life easier for you.

Some governments provide help to buy things like wheelchair ramps, or help in providing funding to make any needed renovations to your house to make things easier for you. In most cases, you would pay part of the amount, and the government the other.

Some governments (e.g. US) have established or authorized some type of program to provide pharmaceutical (as in prescribed medication) coverage for low-income seniors or people with disabilities who do not qualify for Medicaid, or their federal health benefits program.

Many governments will offer income tax relief to people with Parkinson's. You will need to fill out forms to apply for this, but it's definitely worth checking into to see if you qualify for this.

Sometimes, applying for benefits can be complicated, time-consuming, and maybe frustrating. Two things you need to remember when going through this process are: 1) do not throw away any potentially relevant paperwork you receive from an employer, an insurer, a government agency, or an advocate on your behalf and 2) keep copies of everything that you submit.

As was said before, you will need to do some research to find out whether or not you qualify for government assistance. You might start with your local chapter for Parkinson's (check the phone book in yellow or white pages) and they can tell you where you need to go. Depending on what country you live in, you may receive more or less benefits.

How Does the Law Cover People With Parkinson's in Employment?

First and foremost, remember that just because you have Parkinson's does not mean you have lost all (if any) of your rights at your place of work. Don't let any employer tell you differently!

Yes, countries will be different in their laws, but it's important that you find out from your local government officials as to what exactly your rights are as a person with Parkinson's.

One piece of advice Mom found to be very helpful when she was diagnosed with PD and still working, was to go and meet with her Human Resources Department at work right away.

This is done to inform them of your new "condition" and to find out any information they may have to offer you.

It's important that when you go though, you don't go alone. Bring someone with you to take notes and be your "witness" to prevent possible problems down the road.

Is it Safe to Drive if You Have Parkinson's?

Many people think that once they have been diagnosed with Parkinson's they will have to give up driving. This isn't necessarily true. Each case of Parkinson's is different and the disease progresses at a different rate in each person.

Although driving isn't safe in the advanced stages of Parkinson's, people with milder symptoms who can control their impaired motor abilities can continue driving.

There are several issues that are involved in deciding on whether or not you should be driving with your PD. Your physical ability, legal permission, safety, and the importance of keeping your independence all play a part.

You will probably be able to drive safely and legally for several years, depending on your age and general physical condition. However, PD eventually affects reaction time, ability to handle multiple tasks, vision, and judgment.

A good way to figure out whether you should be behind the wheel is to ask yourself, "If a loved one were my passenger, would I be risking that person's safety because of my PD?"

Also, pay attention to how others react to your driving. If your loved ones have said negative things about how you drive or they aren't sure whether or not they want to be your passenger, you may want to think carefully about their concerns.

My mom chooses not to drive most of the time because it causes her to tense up and this causes her muscles to hurt.

BONUS:
55 Real Life Secrets and Practical Tips That Someone With Parkinson's Can Use Every Single Day To Make Their Life Easier, Happier and More Productive

----

BONUS: 55 PRACTICAL TIPS TO MAKE LIFE EASIER WITH PARKINSON'S

FOR YOUR CLOTHING:

1. Wear clothing that you don't have to put on over your head as this will make it easier for you to get dressed.

2. Buy clothing that does up with snaps and not small buttons as you may not have the dexterity to do them up.

3. Wear layers of cool clothing (e.g.. cotton) as you may need to peel them off if you experience dyskinesia which can cause your body temperature to go up.

4. Wear smooth soled shoes to avoid tripping.

5. Buy a watch with big buttons on it so you won't have troubles setting it. (Mom uses her digital watch to keep track of when to take her medications so the big buttons make it a lot easier for her to set it)

6. Get a watchband that does up with Velcro as it is much easier to work with than the buckle kind.

7. Buy shoes and boots that do up with a zipper to help make them easier to get on. Velcro is also good (but maybe not as stylish Mom says)

8. Wear underwear made from slippery fabrics (like satin for women or poly/cotton material men). This can make putting on jeans much faster.

9. Use a dressing stick (a long stick with a hook on the end of it) to help you get dressed while seated. You can use it to grab clothes off the floor or to position them on yourself without straining from reaching or bending.

IN THE BATHROOM:

10. As soon as possible, buy yourself an electric toothbrush. (Mom says this is compulsory!) It can be very hard getting the hand motion going that is needed to brush your teeth with a regular toothbrush.

11. Put a shower wand in the bath tub to make showering much easier and faster.

12. Buy a rubber mat to put in the bath tub to avoid slipping and/or falling.
13. Install handle bars on the side of the tub to help getting in and out. Also,

install grab bars on the shower wall to balance when showering and on the wall beside the toilet.

14. Have a chair in the bathroom so you can sit if you are too tired to stand while brushing your teeth, etc.

15. Buy an inexpensive outdoor chair or bench that is webbed or made of resin to put in the bathtub. This can allow you to sit while showering to avoid slipping and also make it easier on your legs.

IN THE KITCHEN:

16. Buy light weight utensils so they don't fall out of your hands when you're trying to use them. (*this is what works best for my mom, but you will have to see if getting lighter or heavier utensils is better for you)

17. Instead of wearing a bib to catch food droppings, use paper towel that can be clipped on to your shirt with a tie clip (for men) or a scarf clip (for women). Mom doesn't like the idea of wearing a bib. Call it pride or whatever, she just keeps lots of paper towel or napkins and her scarf clip with her whenever she's going somewhere where she might be eating.

18. Try stain resistant clothing as this is a nifty little invention that can save you from having to launder your clothes so much.

19. Concentrate when eating, especially when you are by yourself.

20. To avoid choking when eating, eat with your chin lowered, looking at your food (and not "gawking all over the place", as Mom would say)

21. Stay away from the stove and counters where knives are kept when you have dyskinesia to avoid accidents.

22. To make it easier to grip glasses, fill them halfway, use narrower glasses or try cups or mugs with two handles.

IN THE BEDROOM:

23. Install a pole that stands beside your bed to help you get in and out of it easier. If you can't install a pole because your ceiling is super high, you can install a wooden arm or grab bar on the wall (Mom's is adjustable and is homemade). These devices can also help you turn over in bed.

24. Never use flannelette or t-shirt material sheets. Instead, buy ones with a satin finish to allow you to move more freely in bed (don't forget your pillow cases too).

25. If your bedroom is currently positioned a long way away from the bathroom, you may want to consider moving your bedroom closer to make getting there that much easier (especially in the middle of the night).

26. Keep a container with lid and drinking straw by the bed to sip at during the night.

IN THE LIVING ROOM:

27. Have a "station" where you sit and have as much stuff (ex. medications, water, cane, books, crafts, etc.) as possible that you might need. When you sit down, it may be a while before you get back up again so the more stuff that you have nearby, the better.

28. To avoid slipping and falling, get rid of scatter mats. Also, it is much easier to get around on hardwood or tiled floors than carpet, so you may want to consider replacing your carpets.

29. To get out of your chair, sit on the edge, put your feet underneath the chair, and "launch" yourself out (this sounds funny, but that's basically the way Mom does it). You may need to rock a bit back and forth first in order to gain some momentum.

30. Put some slippery fabric on all of your chairs and couches (and cushions) to make it easier to move around on them.

31. You may find having an office chair on wheels in the house is handy as well. If you have hardwood or tiled floors, you can use this as a makeshift wheelchair for someone to push you from A to B. Mom uses a chair like this at the kitchen table for eating, but can then roll into the living room or bedroom if she wants to as well.

WHEN YOU'RE WALKING:

32. "You don't want heavy grabbers on your feet", Mom says. In other words, you don't want shoes that grip the floor and cause you to stumble.

33. If you are having trouble walking in the house, try taking all of your footwear off. Mom finds that making a bare foot connection with the floor makes it easier for her to walk.

34. Sometimes walking with someone can be better than using a walker. Mom says make sure you (the person with PD) are holding onto them, and not them holding onto you. This will give you more confidence and you get to determine when you want to let go.

35. Make a clear pathway from your bedroom to the bathroom to prevent tripping and falling at night. You may want to install grab bars or a railing along the wall to help guide you, as well as a night light.

36. Here's a neat thing mom discovered recently. Having a contrasting pattern on the floor or ground helps her get from A to B much easier. For example, in the house she had a friend cut out white squares (8 x 8 inches made of vinyl on one side and sticky material on the other) and taped them down to the floor to make a "path" between the kitchen and the bathroom.

When mom needs to go from the kitchen to the bathroom and is having troubles walking, looking down at the contrasting white squares on the floor helps her brain be more focussed on getting to where she wants to be. She has done something similar outside as well. By making a stone pathway (made of pre-cut white patio cement she got at the local hardware store) from the stairs of her house to her garden, she is able to "follow the yellow brick road" (or white in this case) as I like to say it, and get to her garden without any problem.

This tip could be applied to anything, really. If you or your loved one is having mobility problems with PD, having a contrasting pattern put on the floor or ground may be just the answer they need.

WHEN YOU'RE OUT SHOPPING:

37. Use a buggy when shopping if you are feeling at all unstable. If you are by yourself, make sure you have something in the buggy for added weight so you can lean on it if need be.

38. Walkers on wheels are good for a while but if you have problems with freezing, they may not be for you. Mom used to use a walker on wheels but now is unable because her feet won't go as fast as it goes and the breaks aren't fast enough.

39. Most shopping malls have wheelchairs to borrow for the day. Don't be afraid to ask for one if you are feeling tired or unstable. Mom loves to shop and it's not fun when we have to cut the shopping trip short because her legs have shut down. Getting a wheelchair means we can go for the whole day without worrying about if and when she may shutdown.

40. Bring your bank card when shopping. Many stores allow you to use debit cards, which are, as Mom says, the greatest invention. By paying with your bank card, there's no fumbling for change or trying to sign your name for credit cards or cheques. This will avoid any stress you may feel about being slow and holding up the line, etc.

41. Look for automatic doors when going in and out of the store as these are way

easier to go through.

42. Shop at stores with family washrooms where your caregiver can come in with you (if opposite gender). This way your caregiver can take you right to the door of the cubicle, should you need this assistance.

WHEN YOU'RE IN THE CAR:

43. Apply to get a disabled parking permit so you can park in the closer spots.

44. To make getting in and out of the car easier (if your car does not have leather or vinyl seats) put a piece of slippery fabric on the seat (you can even use a garbage bag).

45. Keep an extra water bottle (and a straw if you use them) and crackers in the car to take medications with.

46. Keep an extra outfit in the car in case you spill something and need to change.

47. Have an extra pillow or two in the car for long trips to keep you as comfortable as possible.

WHEN TAKING YOUR MEDICATIONS:

48. Buy a digital sports watch that has a countdown repeat timer to keep track of when you need to take your medications. Mom has one of these that she sets to beep every 3 hours to remind her to take her meds.

49. Make a daily medication list and tape it to your fridge. We actually made and printed one up for mom on the computer that has the whole day planned out for her. (For example, at 6:30 am she takes 1 Sinemet Control Release and 3 Mirapex, at 9:30 am she takes 1 Sinemet, 1 Selegiline and 1 Mirapex, etc.)

50. Use a weekly pill organizer that has slots for each day. Fill the organizer at the beginning of each week.

WHEN YOU'RE WRITING:

51. Buy pencils and pens that have wide grips because they are easy to hold onto and use.

52. Use pen or pencil grips to help you keep hold of them. These are small

cylinder shaped pieces of rubber with a hole in the center that you put your pen or pencil through. It will stay in place until you move it or take it off.

53. Try twisting a rubber band around a pen or pencil several times to help you keep your grip.

54. If you are having difficulties writing, try printing instead as this may be easier for you.

55. If you like to use the computer a lot but find it hard to type, there is software called "Via Voice" that you can buy that is very affordable. This software allows you to talk into your computer through a headset microphone and it writes down what you are saying.

The program can be taught to understand different peoples' voices so that you and anybody else who is using your computer might use it. It is a great tool!

EXTRA BONUS TIPS: SOME OF THE MOST VALUABLE THINGS YOU SHOULD KNOW TO HELP WITH PARKINSON'S

1. Music is Very Powerful

It took almost fifteen years with the disease for my mom to find out the power of music. She says it was a total surprise to find out how effective it was in getting her mobilized the first time she tried it.

What she did was when she was having an "off" period, she played some upbeat music that she liked and in a matter of a few minutes (and now sometimes in a few seconds) she was up and moving.

When we (her kids) found out about this, we suggested she buy an MP3 player to carry with her anywhere she went. This way she could play the music ANYTIME she found her "wheels" (her legs) were shutting down.

"An MP3 player", she said, "what's that?" We explained to her that instead of playing audio tapes or CDs, it plays from an electronic file called an MP3 (you can get your favourite songs put onto it through your computer or ask someone you know to do it for you).

This allows it to be quite small, and in fact, Mom's is the size of a lipstick container. She loves it! She has it hung around her neck during the day and "plugs in" whenever she needs to.

A CD player would work as well, except Mom liked the idea of it being so small that it could hang around her neck to get at it easily, and the fact that she doesn't have to fumble around to put the CD's in.

It really is AMAZING to watch Mom when she literally is stuck in place and after putting on her music, she can motor anywhere!

2. Exercise is Very Important

You hear it all the time, whether you have PD or not, that exercising regularly is important. Well, Mom says this has proven to be very important in her life.

Just the simple act of getting outside once a day to go for a walk or putter around can loosen up her muscles, and diminish any depression she might be experiencing.

Exercise (like walking) is also very helpful for her when she is experiencing dyskinesia, as it tends to lessen it almost immediately.

One other reason Mom recommends exercising is because it's good for your lungs which are affected by PD and may need more exercise than others who don't have PD. Singing is also recommended for exercising the lungs.

3. Stress is BAD!

You've probably heard that stress is bad, but it's really bad for people with Parkinson's.

Mom is very aware of how debilitating (ie. how it can cause your body to basically shutdown) stress can be and tries to avoid it if at all possible (she tries, but we all know it's sometimes easier said than done).

She says the more she can focus on doing what's good for her (and not be worried or stressed about the things going on around her) the better things are and the better she feels. The bottom line is, avoid stress!

4. Help is Available

There are many people that will help you if you need it, Mom says. Even when you don't ask for it, people will offer to help you.

Mom is often asked if she would like help with her groceries, or if she would like an arm to hold onto if she is having troubles walking.

Sometimes people don't know if you want help so they may avoid asking you. "You don't have to feel like you're going to be stuck." Mom says, "Ask for help".

5. The Importance of a Good Doctor

Mom has often said how important it has been for her to have a good relationship with her doctor. She can talk to her doctor about anything anytime.

She is never stressed or worried at what he might say when she asks him questions. "You have to feel at ease around your doctor" she says. "You need to be able to tell him or her exactly what's happening with you on a daily basis, so that he/she can adjust your medications along the way".

BONUS:
A Helpful Guide For Parkinson's Caregivers:
14 Vital Tips To Help You Care For The Person You Know Or Love

----

BONUS: A HELPFUL GUIDE FOR PARKINSON'S CAREGIVERS: 14 VITAL TIPS TO HELP YOU CARE FOR THE PERSON YOU KNOW OR LOVE

----

1. Take One Day at a Time

Being a caregiver is or can be a 24 hour, 7 days a week, 365 days a year job. Because of this, one of the biggest challenges you will face is being very tired. Your life can also be very challenging and frustrating because the time you have to yourself is limited.

In addition to this, because the progression of Parkinson's disease is so unpredictable it makes planning for the future very hard. Taking things one day at a time makes it easier to live each day to the fullest. It reduces the stress levels of the person with PD as they don't have to worry about whether or not they will be able to do this or that in the future.

2. Patience Goes a Long Way

One of the most important things a caregiver needs when dealing with someone with Parkinson's is patience.

Being patient is sometimes easier said than done, but a caregiver needs to be aware that his or her stress levels can and do affect a person with PD in a negative way.

Making negative comments of any type as well as giving an angry look can be picked up a person with PD and make their symptoms worse.

One way to increase your patience as a caregiver is to remind yourself that it is the disease, and not the person that is frustrating you.

3. Respite Care is a MUST

A respite worker is someone who can come into your home and help a person with PD with activities of daily living, etc. This gives the caregiver a break from having to do this everyday which can lead to burnout.

Depending on how much care the person with PD needs on a daily basis, the caregiver may chose to take one or more days "off" a week from care giving and have a respite worker come in. Dave (my mom's husband and caregiver) finds that taking one day off a week works well for him.

As a caregiver it's important that you not feel guilty about wanting to have time off and have a respite worker come in. It is not selfish for you to want this time off. Rather, it is absolutely NECESSARY that you do take it, both for your sake and the person you are taking care of.

"People feel that I'm running away", Dave says, but you're not. You're just stepping back off the playing field for a little bit and giving yourself a break. It can also be a good break for the person with PD.

Remember that burnout can come easily and without the caregiver being able to function means the person with PD won't be functioning either.

4. Educate Yourself

When Dave first met my mom, he had no idea what Parkinson's was and what it meant for her to have it. He says it's very important to know what you're dealing with so you know what to do and what to expect.

Dave is a firm believer in education. He says that educating himself about PD has been one of the most important things he has done as a caregiver.

5. Try a Caregiver Group

Caregiver groups are important but you need to be careful that you find one that is upbeat and positive. "Some care groups can be nothing more than a bunch of people whining and complaining and this can make you feel more depressed", Dave says.

It is also important that you make sure the group has a caring and compassionate facilitator who can make sure that the group stays on track.

Finally, when you are at the caregiver group, be careful to never speak out negatively about the person you are caring for, and keep your complaints related to the disease.

6. A Person with PD Can Make Life Easier for the Caregiver

Even though most of the "jobs" are for the caregiver, there are some things that the person receiving the care can do to make things easier.

First of all, it is important that the person with PD be very supportive of the caregiver taking time off to be alone.

Second, whenever possible the person with PD should try to do things on their own without the caregiver's assistance.

Third, it is important for the care receiver to realize that the caregiver has a frustrating and challenging job and they should not take it personally if and when the caregiver is feeling frustrated or upset.

Finally, though it may sound a little contradictory, it is important to make life easier for the caregiver so he or she can then make life easier for the person with PD.

7. Parkinson's Does Not Have to Come Between You and Your Loved One

If you are a caregiver you probably have a close relationship with the person you are caring for. Whether it's your spouse, your mother or father, friend or other relative, it's very important for you both to realize that the problems you are facing are not from the person, but the disease.

Parkinson's is a disease that could come between the two of you, and you have to be careful not to let it. You have to find things that you can still do together or find new things that you both can enjoy.

Whether it's watching TV or whatever, you have to find ways of doing things together that are fun and not a struggle for the person with PD and that don't require patience on the part of the caregiver.

"It can be very easy to lose the relationship you have with one another and just become the caregiver and care receiver. You lose the sense of being a man and a woman, of being husband and wife, of lovers, of companions and friends", Dave says.

"You need to make a very concerted effort to do the types of things to maintain that sense of relationship above and beyond being a caregiver and care receiver".

8. Watch those Meds

Taking medications is a part of every day life for people with Parkinson's. There are several ways to keep track of your medications such as a pill box, a watch with a timer, a chart on the fridge, etc. As a caregiver, it is also important that you monitor whether or not your loved one has taken their medications.

Mom uses a watch with a timer but sometimes she forgets to reset the watch after she has taken the meds, or sometimes when her watch beeps to remind her to take the meds she is in the middle of something and then forgets to take them later.

By keeping track of when Mom is supposed to take her medications, Dave can remind her if need be, meaning no missed meds for Mom.

9. Be a Cheerleader!

One of the greatest, most helpful things you can do for someone you are caring for that has Parkinson's is to be their cheerleader. There are many struggles that a person with PD must face in any given day and having someone by their side to encourage and give them support can be incredibly valuable.

People with PD may need encouragement for many things such as going through doorways, walking, getting up from a chair, eating, or when they are feeling depressed.

Mom especially appreciates the encouragement when she is having difficulties walking, and also really appreciates hugs when she's feeling down. It may not seem like much, but a few kind words or a gentle touch can really make a difference in the life of a person with PD.

10. Take a Coffee Break

As mentioned before in tip #3 about having respite care, it is essential that the caregiver take a break from care giving to avoid burnout.

This may mean having a whole day off when a respite worker comes into your house. It may also mean that when you are caring for someone all day long, you take small breaks.

These breaks should be scheduled ahead of time, so that the person with PD knows you will not be available for short periods of time throughout the day.

For example, Dave says at the beginning of each day he will tell Mom that he'll be taking 2 to 3 breaks that day and gives her an approximate time that he would like to have the breaks. Before he goes for his break, Dave makes sure Mom has everything she needs so that she won't have to call for him to get her something.

Obviously, Dave tries to schedule the breaks when it's convenient for both of them and reassures Mom that he won't just up and leave at the moment he is to have his break if Mom needs him at that moment.

Taking short breaks during the day is very important as they can give the caregiver a chance to recharge and be able to make it through the day with far less frustration and fatigue.

11. Offer Suggestions

Often times you may find the person you are caring for getting frustrated because they are unable to complete certain daily activities that they once were able to.

One common area of frustration is walking. Depending on the stage of Parkinson's that they are in, you may be able to help a person with PD overcome some of their difficulties.

For example, Mom often has trouble walking when her meds are starting to wear off. Often times when this is happening, she starts to get frustrated and forgets that she knows other ways of getting from A to B.

Here's where the caregiver can jump in and offer some suggestions to help her out. What Dave does is he simply suggests to Mom, "Why don't you try walking sideways, Val?" Mom does, and immediately she is on her way.

It's important that Dave not tell Mom what to do, but suggest or ask her if she'd like to try another method of walking. This way Mom is still choosing on her own as to what she would like to do, and doesn't feel ordered around.

12. Do the Locomotion...

Well, it's kind of like the locomotion. What I'm talking about is when Mom is tired, her meds are wearing off and she is having a lot of troubles walking.

Dave has her stand behind him and put her arms around his waist. He then says something like "Left, Right, Left, Right..." to get her started and they essentially become a train going from one place to the next.

This may not be practical in public, but both Mom and Dave find it very useful in the house when other ways of getting around aren't working.

13. Have Stations Around the House

By stations I mean areas in the house where the person you are caring for has everything they may need to spend up to several hours at a time without requiring too much assistance from you the caregiver.

For example, if they spend a lot of time in the living room, you may want to create an area in this room where all the things they may need or like to use are in one place.

A station in the living room might include books, remote controls, water, medications, snacks, knitting, pillows, blankets, etc. Having a "station" where they have all the stuff they may need for several hours makes it so that you as a caregiver don't have to keep getting up to get them things.

14. **Don't Panic!**

Getting ready to go out for the weekend, day, or even for just a few hours for an appointment can be very stressful for both the person with PD and the caregiver. The good news is that much of this stress can be prevented by planning ahead.

It is easy to forget that it can take much longer than you, for a person with PD to get ready. As a caregiver, the first thing you need to be is patient. Remember that getting stressed out about being on time will only make the person you are caring for stressed and this could end the trip before it even starts.

The second thing you can do is done the night before. No matter what the length of trip, there is always some preparation that can be done beforehand.

Getting things together in one place so you both know where to find them in the morning helps you avoid having to run around looking for things five minutes before you are supposed to leave.

BONUS:
Pain and Parkinson's Disease: Answers to Common Questions

BONUS: PAIN AND PARKINSON'S DISEASE: ANSWERS TO COMMON QUESTIONS

----

1. Is pain common in Parkinson's?

Yes, pain is quite common in PD. It is said that up to 40 to 50 percent of people with Parkinson's disease experience pain. Many times people with PD don't realize the impact that pain has on their condition because symptoms like stiffness, tremor, falls and dyskinesia may be more obvious to them.

Sometimes pain can be the main symptom of Parkinson's, so it's important that both people with Parkinson's and their caregivers be aware of the problems pain may cause in Parkinson's.

2. What are the types and causes of pain in PD?

There are various different types of pain in Parkinson's disease, all with their own causes. Recently, researchers have tried to classify these types of pain which are listed below.

Musculoskeletal Pain:

This is a common type of pain in Parkinson's. It starts from muscles and bone and you will usually feel it as an ache around your joints, arms and legs.

The pain stays in one place and does not move around or "shoot" down a leg or arm. This type of pain is caused by the muscle rigidity in PD which leads to cramps and spasms.

Mom has a lot of experience with this type of pain. She frequently has hip butt, and calf pains and spasms. To help with the pain, she sees a massage therapist regularly who massages the area for about 20 minutes to get rid of the pain. The therapist then gives mom specific exercises for stretching the tightened muscles which she can also do at home.

Radicular Pain:

This type of pain is a sharp, shooting pain that can feel like a shock that travels down a leg or an arm and may be felt in your fingers and toes. You may often feel tingling and numbness or a burning feeling in your toes and/or fingers.

This type of pain is usually the result of a trapped nerve inside the spinal cord around the neck or back area. Nerves could be trapped by protruding "discs" which normally act as "pillows" between the bony vertebrae or due to arthritis of the spine.

Dyskinetic Pain:

If you have dyskenisia (abnormal involuntary movements) with your PD, you may experience this type of pain. This type of pain can happen in the daytime either before, during or after the dyskinesias. Sometimes, people with Parkinson's feel body pain as dyskinesias are about to start, so the pain could be a kind of warning sign for the dyskinesias.

Dyskinetic pain can happen anywhere on the body and can feel like an aching pain. Some people with Parkinson's feel pain during severe dyskinesias, perhaps because of the twisting movements. Also, dyskinesias can make radicular pain worse if you have a trapped nerve underneath.

You may also feel this type of pain because of changing responses to PD medications, like Levodopa. As you experience changes in your responses to the drugs, you may experience something called dystonia early in the morning or late at night. This is when you get a spasm in parts of your body like your fingers, wrists, toes or ankles.

Dystonia can happen when your drugs are wearing off at night and can do things like cause your feet to turn inwards. Because it can feel like a painful cramp, dystonia may even wake you up early in the morning.

Akathisia:

This is when you have a sense of restlessness that causes pain. This kind of pain can often happen at night and you may find it hard to sleep because you fidget in bed and want to move your arms and legs.

Akathisia can happen as result of taking certain drugs for Parkinson's. This pain is also hard to describe and feels more like discomfort instead of pain. This discomfort usually involves the legs and if you get it, you may find yourself wandering around trying to get relief from it.

3. Are there any other types of pain in PD?

There are sometimes different kinds of pain that happen in Parkinson's that are different from the kinds of pain described above. These types of pain are described below:

Shoulder, Arm, and Leg Pain:

Sometimes pain and stiffness on one side of your body, usually an arm or leg, can be the first sign that you are developing Parkinson's. When this happens, your doctor may refer you to someone who specializes in conditions affecting the joints (called a rheumatologist) and a diagnosis for Parkinson's may be mistakenly delayed.

This type of pain is constant, and feels like an ache. You will find that your ability to do fine movements with your fingers will be decreased or that you start dragging a foot. If the pain remains constant, continues to ache, and the arm or leg becomes more and more stiff, Parkinson's may be suspected.

Burning Mouth:

Although it is rare and unusual, some people with PD experience a burning sensation or pain in their mouth. This can happen at any stage of Parkinson's and researchers are unsure of the cause.

One study has said that this type of pain in the mouth might affect up to 24 percent of people with Parkinson's. Some say that dry mouth caused by certain drugs taken for PD (like benzhexol) as well as dentures that don't fit properly may be responsible.

Coat Hanger Pain:

This is a rare type of pain that is sometimes seen in people with Parkinson's who also have something called postural hypotension (when your blood pressure drops as soon as you stand up). However, this type of pain is more common in people who have a form of Parkinson's called Multiple System Atrophy (MSA) rather than Parkinson's.

Coat hanger pain will usually start around the back of your neck and sometimes move to the back of your head and shoulder muscles. It is called coat hanger pain because the overall shape of the area of the body where the pain is looks like a coat hanger.

Researchers aren't sure of the cause of this type of pain but some think that it may occur due to reduced blood supply (due to postural hypotension) to the muscles in the neck and shoulder area.

Akinetic Crisis Pain:

If your PD symptoms suddenly get worse, this may have happened as a result of suddenly stopping your Parkinson's treatment or by infections.

The symptoms of this type of pain include severe stiffness, fever, pain in muscles and joints, headaches, and sometimes, whole body pain. Severe stiffness in the muscles causing the release of pain producing chemicals may be the cause.

Headache:

By headache we mean head pain. This kind of pain can happen at any stage in people with Parkinson's and sometimes can be caused by the drugs used to treat Parkinson's (for example the dopamine agonists amantadine and entacapone).

Muscle Cramps:

People with PD can experience muscle cramps that may come on during the night or day. At night they may cause pain in the legs and calf muscles as well as restlessness, which causes you to lose sleep.

Cramps in Parkinson's can also happen when the effect of drugs (ex. Levodopa) is wearing off. This cramping can be painful and may happen as a result of an involuntary contraction of your muscles.

You can get cramps in internal organs with muscles as well which will affect your bowel (causing abdominal pain and cramps) or bladder (making it painful to urinate or having an urgency to urinate).

4. How can you treat pain in PD?

In order to treat pain in PD successfully, you need to know the **cause** of the pain. Some treatments are listed below:

Musculoskeletal Pain:

This type of pain may respond to a combination of painkillers such as paracetamol along with regular exercise, massage therapy and physiotherapy.

Radicular Pain:

If you experience this type of pain, you should talk to your doctor about it. You may find out that you need an X-ray of the affected area. In most cases simple painkillers and regular, light exercise will be enough to treat it.

Though it doesn't happen very often, if you have this pain severe enough and it won't go away, you may need a referral to a neurologist to rule out compression of the nerve roots at your spinal cord.

The neurologist may have you take magnetic resonance imaging (MRI) scans and may ask you to wear a neck collar if the problem arises from your neck.

Dyskinetic Pain:

This pain is mostly related to "off" periods (when you find it difficult to be mobile) when your Parkinson's drugs are wearing off. If you can make the "on" period (when the anti-Parkinson's drugs are effective) last longer, then you can help this kind of pain.

To do this, try taking small and frequent doses of levodopa drugs, combining levodopa with a COMT inhibitor such as entacapone or using a long acting dopamine agonist drug, such as cabergoline. Sometimes night-time "off" related pain may also be helped by taking a long-acting drug, such as cabergoline, at night.

There's a drug called apomorphine that can help you if your "off" period pain is caused by early morning dystonia (remember, this is when you get a spasm in a group of muscles). If your body doesn't respond to the self injections of the apomorphine, your doctor may suggest drug called botulinum toxin that can also be taken through injections.

Occasionally, dyskinesia-related pain can happen when your PD meds are working well (in other words, before they start to wear off) and in these cases the doses of relevant drugs will have to be reduced. When you have pain that is related to your dyskinesia, you need to talk to your neurologist to get the proper help.

Akathisia:

If you feel this type of pain at night, you will often find that you can help relieve it by combining your medications for PD that you take at night, such as controlled release levodopa (or long acting dopamine agonist drug) together with meds that can help you sleep, like amitriptyline or zopiclone.

Shoulder, Arm, and Leg Pain:

You may be able to help these types of pain if your regular PD medications are helping control your PD. You can also try seeing a physiotherapist as they can be helpful as well.

My mom has had both shoulder and leg pain and sees a massage therapist, physiotherapist, and occasionally an acupuncturist for these which have all been helpful.

If you continue to feel pain, you may need painkillers, and should talk to your doctor as well as you may need a referral to a specialist in this area.

Burning Mouth:

If you have this type of pain, you should be referred to a dentist. Rinsing out your mouth regularly with an antiseptic mouthwash and keeping your mouth moist with drinks are also important. You may find that sucking on a piece of ice may also be helpful in hot weather.

If you have dentures that don't fit properly, you need to remove them. Also, if you are being treated with drugs such as benzhexol, talk to your doctor as you may need to discontinue their use as such drugs can cause dry mouth.

Coat Hanger Pain:

If you have this type of pain, you need to talk to your doctor and ask for a referral to a specialist who has experience with movement disorders so you can get a proper diagnosis and treatment.

Akinetic Crisis Pain:

You can usually help this by taking levodopa drugs.

Headaches:

Because headaches in people with PD aren't often very severe, over the counter painkillers are usually enough to stop the pain. You should be careful not to take too many pills at once though, especially if you are taking medication for high blood pressure or heart problems.

You should try to space out all the pills you are taking as much as possible because if you take them all together, they may cause headaches. Although it doesn't happen very often, if you have a severe headache that won't go away, you should talk to a neurologist.

Muscle Cramps:

You will often find that your PD medications can help with muscle cramps. For example, if you get cramps at night, you can help them by making levodopa last longer by taking the controlled release version of the drug. You may also want to try taking soluble levodopa dissolved in fizzy orange juice.

In some situations, when there is severe 'off' period-related bowel cramps, apomorphine injections may be very helpful.

Some tonic waters contain quinine which is often prescribed for cramps in tablet form and may help if taken at night. Just make sure you check that the brand of tonic water you use does contain quinine (ex. Schweppes) because not all of them do. The drug diazepam may sometimes be useful too.

5. Where can I get help for my pain?

First of all, you need to let your doctor or neurologist know about the problem. Usually your doctor will be able to manage the more common types of pain such as musculoskeletal, shoulder pain and headaches.

However, certain other types of pain such as dyskinetic pain, burning mouth or coat hanger pain may need referral to a neurologist who has experience in Parkinson's disease treatment.

Bonus Tips to Help With Pain in PD:

----

1. If you are taking pain medications, be aware that some of them can cause constipation so you may need to be more diligent in your anti-constipation routine.

2. Keep extra pillows and cushions handy on the couch and on your bed to place between or under your knees, or back, or wherever you need them to make you more comfortable.

3. When you are in pain and you want to sleep, finding the position that's comfortable may take some time and a fair bit of movement. This is why it's very important that you have "slippery" bed sheets and night clothing. Also, a grab bar at the side of the bed can be a big help to help you find that comfortable position as well.

MAKING LIFE WITH PARKINSON'S EASIER

MORE THAN 199 TIPS, ADVICE, STORIES, AND WORDS OF ENCOURAGEMENT AND INSPIRATION FROM PEOPLE WITH PARKINSON'S ALL OVER THE WORLD

Lianna Marie

CONTENTS

TIPS FROM A TO Z

ALTERNATIVE TREATMENTS

"At this stage, (my Parkinson's is in the early stage with a shaking in my left hand and foot) I find a great benefit from meditation. I listen to the program for 1 hour a day, usually at bedtime, and I become super relaxed and sleep all night without problems.

I use CD's from Centerpointe Research Institute and all the information is on their website at www.centerpointe.com"

- Ken from Queensland, Australia

"I am from India (currently residing in Canada) and my mother has Parkinson's (she lives in India).

It is amazing to note that there have been not one, but two alternative cures, all outside the known medical world, that have been offered to my mother. And I must say they are all harmless and do not cost much money.

How much these improve the condition is very difficult to say. I am sure that it will vary from one person to another, but seeing it on my mother I think I would certainly say that they have positive effects, and nothing negative.

I am not selling these ideas to anyone here, just sharing my views, and I do not want anyone to blindly believe what I am saying. These are just my own personal views with no scientific proof or base to them.

The remedies that I have found are.....

1. Reiki - This is touch therapy. I am sure you will find lots on the internet about this. My mother tried this, and the day of her first session with the Reiki expert she almost immediately felt relieved. Even the next day morning she was feeling much better, and this was just after 1 sitting. She had 2 more sittings after that, but how this will really benefit her in the long run after the total treatment is over, is still to be seen.

2. Yoga - There are a few institutes in India (as I'm sure there must be in other parts of the world too), that offer full time yoga courses. Some of these even claim to have cured cancer patients, and it is just by disciplined and very

dedicated yoga sessions that cures happen. My mother has not yet tried this out, but we are hoping that she will go for it in the near future.

The reason that I write this is to give people some hope outside the medical world. There may be alternative remedies that can cure or at least reduce the effect of Parkinson's, and we shouldn't lose hope."

- Rohit

"I have two things to try. One is glutathione patches distributed by LifeWave Products. Dr. Perlmuter from Florida really believes in glutathione. It is usually injected. The other thing is gene therapy which I can do at Oregon Health Sciences in Portland."

- Mary Ellen

"When I looked up Parkinson's disease on the internet last spring, I had not even been diagnosed. That week I made my 30th appointment with my doctor and came right out and asked him if my balance disorder, posture and gait could be Parkinson's and I also told him that my grandmother had it. He said absolutely no, that I had nothing neurological wrong. He said it was sodalities in my back.

With great relief, I read no more about Parkinson's, and asked the doctor to refer me to a back specialist. He did, but it was going to take eight months before I could see the specialist. In the mean time I was getting more bent, and basically I sat all day and just moved from one chair to the next.
Finally summer came and my daughter and family arrived from Ireland. What a shock they got when I met them at the airport, as they had not seen me since Christmas.

At the end of August they returned back to Ireland, and my daughter was so upset about my condition that she emailed her best friend in Toronto whose father is head of Orthopedics.

To make a long story short, we found out that Spondylitis never causes a balance problem, and that I needed to be seen by a neurologist. Reluctantly my family doctor sent me to see one on September the 6th, and I was diagnosed with Parkinson's in a New York minute.

I am on Sinemet and Comtan. The meds worked a bit, but I was still not great, though better for sure than I was.

After two months on the drugs a very good friend of mine told me a story of her husband, who fell ill for years. He visited every doctor in Toronto, and took every pill but he just continued to be no better. As a last kick at the cat, my friend was given a card of a Chinese herbalist in Toronto. Together with his wife they decided they had nothing to lose, and to visit the man.

After six months of drinking special teas made for him, he was back to work and today has never looked back. He told me that if he was ever diagnosed with a chronic illness he would most definitely pay the Chinese doctor a visit and felt I should.

Like this man, I felt I had nothing to lose. I phoned the Chinese doctor and asked him if he had ever worked with Parkinson's. He told me yes, and though he couldn't cure it, he could definitely make a change for the better.

I went up to Ontario and made my appointment. We talked about balance and posture, really my only complaint, along with the use of a cane.

To make this short, I feel like the disease is gone. My posture has lifted up. I can stand in one spot, and walk long distances with no cane. Friends and family can't believe what's happened in such a short time.

I am able to wear heels again and I am living a normal life. The tea was specially made for me out of very strong Korean Ginseng and other ingredients. I take two a day for one month and then will go to one, and then 3 or 4 a week, after which the doctor will see me again to follow my progress. Perhaps thousands of others could be helped like me."

- Dorothy Fendley from Halifax, Nova Scotia, Canada

"Have you heard about the BPM (Blood Pressure Modulation) therapy machine?

Check website www.bpmtherapy.com

It's very interesting and I want my wife (who has PD) to try it."

- George

"I just can't pretend to give you my advice, but I'll try to let you know my point of view, or at least part of it, relating to Parkinson's.

First of all, a couple of years ago I downloaded an e-book written by Mr. Noel N Batten, an Australian therapist. It was called "Parkinson's Disease - The Greatest Medical Blunder".

As far as Mr. Batten is concerned "Parkinson's disease is nothing more than a stress response to mental over activity causing excessive tension in the neck, lungs and stomach." I wish I had come across that book a few years before! But still I work the four points mentioned by Mr. Batten:

1) Overcoming my overactive mind
2) Exercising my lungs
3) Relaxing my neck muscles
4) Relaxing my stomach muscles

Mr. Batten insists on the importance of R.E.M. sleep, since this is the time when our body regenerates.

That's why I meditate, I see a chiropractor regularly to have vertebrae fixed, especially in the neck. I also work on the possible causes of my over active mind: grief, anxiety, internal conflicts, fear, grudge, etc. that I have kept inside over the years.

Anyway, last year I was given a couple of books by my kid brother. They were written by Dr. Daniel Dufour, a Swiss physician for 25 years. Dr. Dufour points roughly in the same direction: for him any illness, disease or health problem is a message sent by our body, indicating to us that there is an internal conflict that has to be settled, if we want to heal. If you don't explode (exteriorise your problem), you will implode (get sick or ill, or develop some health problems)!! Your weak point will be hit. By the way, Dr. Dufour is on the web.

As for myself, I believe I developed Parkinson's since I had a skull fracture when I was two years of age. And, as you know, statistics show that people that have had a skull injury are four times more susceptible to have Parkinson's.

So to sum up, I think I can't pretend to give too much advice. One last point: a few months ago I came across an article on the wed site of Dr. Joseph Mercola revealing that the correction of upper neck injuries might help improve or even reverse the progression of Multiple Sclerosis and Parkinson's disease!"

- Jean Lépine

"My dear friend has Parkinson's so it has sparked my 'research gene' into action. When I came upon the following website through a recommendation of a coworker I had to try it out. It seemed too good (too simple) to be true.

Well, I was in for the surprise of my life. The technique, when done properly, does everything the site says it will and more. It has not failed to be effective with any situation. I have tested it on things from anger management to bi-polar depression, to fear of snakes. Flu symptoms, headaches, overweight, sexual abuse, hiatus hernia, H.B.P., lack of focus and concentration, and cancer etc., etc. have all been tested and have shown results.

The techniques are available on the site and are FREE. No one has to incur any cost unless they wish to have someone do the work for them instead of doing it themselves. There are also thousands of case histories to read on almost every malady imaginable.

Please take a moment to check this out. You could have just found a major breakthrough in living with the Big 'P'."

www.emofree.com/parkinsons-disease.htm

- Elisabeth Denaro from Phoenix, Arizona, USA

BALANCE

"I have found this to be true with me. If you fall, do not get up right away. Get your feet in order, your hands too. Then think about what and where your next move is going to be, when you are ready get up, and if there is any one around to help you. Tell them to let you be for a minute or two then you will be glad to let them know when they can help you up."

- Jo from North Fort Myers, Florida, USA

"Recently I read on a web site about the benefits of MBT footwear for Parkinson's sufferers. I got a pair for my mother who has had it for about 5 years and she is delighted with them, they assist with balance and are recommended for motor neuron diseases."

Check out: www.mbt-ireland.com Also: www.swissmasaius.com

- Irene

BATHROOM

"For brushing my teeth I use an electric toothbrush but I have difficulty flossing. The answer for me was the Hummingbird battery-operated flosser."

- Anonymous

"The advice I had from our Occupational Therapist was to have a walk-in shower installed, and "Grab Rails" fitted in the bathtub for my husbands' safety."

- Joy

"One subject matter that seems to be avoided as much as possible and I do not know how to say this politely in a genteel fashion, is going to the bathroom.

One changes from being a regular visitor to the bathroom, usually daily with fiber and 5 fruits and vegetables, to an irregular visit. And when you gotta go, you gotta go.

It changes from being a normal stool where the muscles in the intestines shape it, to a paste like substance and lots of it. One can literally block the toilet, no kidding.

I do not know how but I still travel a lot in my job around Europe and so far no accidents. I must have a lucky charm.
One piece of advice for at work is to get an office close to the bathroom. I used to have an office 250 feet from the toilets at work. It is very uncomfortable walking that distance and feeling almost out of control.
So there, I have got it off my chest.

One other thing, do not let oneself get into a poor functioning state physically, especially in the early years. Get on the medicine and do not put it off too long. I, like most, prefer not to acknowledge its progression and prefer to put off the next medicine regime as long as possible. I did and was having difficulty holding down a responsible technical managers' job.

Finally, a problem shared is a problem halved. Let others know, they will come to your aid when needed. Yesterday on an international teleconference I choked on a drink of water. A colleague immediately helped me recover outside the room, without fuss."

- Brian

BEDROOM

"The bedside rail has been a wonderful tool. My mother hasn't slipped off the side of the bed since we purchased the rail."

- Anonymous

CAREGIVING

"Living with Parkinson's disease can be overwhelming. My husband was diagnosed about 5 years ago although we think that he has had it longer. Today he is 62 years old.

When he was first diagnosed, we were both frightened by what lay ahead for us. It was all an uncharted course for us. I made my husband promise me that he would not give up and that he would cooperate with me as I tried to help him.

He has kept that promise and I believe that it has drawn us closer. We have good days and days when he has a hard time. On the bad days, we just blame "Parky" for his troubles.

Keeping a sense of humor is VITAL!! This disease will overwhelm you if you let it! We laughed when our grandson said, "Grandpa quivers" to which his cousin said "No, his is just shivering".

- Anonymous

"My husband is still able to drive and get around pretty well. He does however, have trouble with dressing, grooming, and cutting his food. Mostly anything that requires hand and finger coordination has become difficult if not impossible.

Here again, he is not too proud to ask for help. The grandchildren are eager to help Grandpa get up from his chair or hand him something. No one treats him like an invalid but each one with "lend a hand" as he needs it.

One thing that I personally feel is SO IMPORTANT is to keep active. With the medications that are given to "manage" Parkinson's, comes a host of side-effects, number one being extreme tiredness. My husband would sit in his recliner and sleep ALL DAY if I let him.

He still takes Carbidopa/Levadopa however he was not able to "tolerate" the "side-effects" from any of the other medications the doctor tried. So, we have turned to a more "natural" approach using Nutritional supplements.

We have found that O.P.C.-3 and CoQ10 along with a good multivitamin and B-12 has really helped him. He takes these supplements in an isotonic form which means that they are absorbed and not digested so he gets about 98% of their value.

We have also learned that (at least in his case) the cold weather really affects him.

The cold and damp weather makes his body very "stiff" and he has more trouble "locking".

"Locking", is another problem when we travel. We have learned that we must plan ahead as getting "locked" in a small place (like the plane's bathroom!) is not good!

For the caregiver/spouse, I offer this advice. Remember, this is the same person you married. He/she is just locked into a body that doesn't work like it used to.

Don't take yourself so seriously. LAUGH together. Parkinson's is just a disease. It doesn't define who you are. It is a good "excuse" for getting a Handicap Parking Card. Look at the bright side, if you take your husband shopping with you, you get great parking!!

You also need some alone time to "recharge your batteries". Don't feel that you have to carry this alone. Involve your family, help each other. Being the caregiver is hard work.

Don't be ashamed if you get tired. It is important that you talk to each other. Just because your mate has Parkinson's doesn't mean that they can't support you emotionally. It is the "body" that doesn't work not the brain and heart!
I sincerely hope that what we have learned will help someone else "cope". How well you "survive" this disease, depends largely on your attitudes. It is a lot easier when you stay positive.

Look for reasons to be happy. Focus on what you CAN still do, not on what you can't! Some days might feel like "a trip downhill" but you can still enjoy the scenery around you on the way! The next day might be better so don't give up!"

- Melody Hodge from Escondido, California, USA

"I drive as often as I can on a weekend to see my friend who has Parkinson's. It's at least an hour's drive each way, since he and his wife moved to be near their son and his young family of four children in case of emergencies.

Both his son and his wife both work hard and are very much involved with their children's activities and their church, so they aren't able to help my friend as much as they'd like.

My friend is 76 and has stage 4 Parkinson's. His wife has suffered dreadfully from rheumatoid arthritis for many years and struggles to cope. Unfortunately, every time he has been offered help by the social services my friend airily replies, "That's all right; we can cope!" much to his wife's justifiable irritation.

When I go to visit he 'takes me to lunch', meaning that I drive us somewhere and he pays for a meal. This gives his wife a very welcome break, so that she can go off and visit a friend for the day, catch up on her sleep or do whatever she wants without having to worry about my friend.

On one of our outings I took the opportunity of gently asking my friend how he would manage if anything happened to his wife. I told him that every woman needs a little time to herself for a bit of rest and relaxation and suggested that he might wish to give his wife time to 'recharge her batteries' by taking advantage of any help that was offered to him.

I am pleased to say that my friend now goes to a day center twice a week where he has lunch and sometimes enjoys the mental exercise of an informal quiz afterwards or recalling the words of an old song.

He has home visits from the nurse on a regular basis, which is also helpful. I guess my tip is to accept help when it is offered, if not for yourself then for your carer's sake. The outcome can give your life more structure and even something to look forward to, which in itself can help disperse some of the depression that comes with the condition."

- Christine

"My aunt is 82 years old and lives next door to me. One of the most difficult parts in caring for my aunt was not allowing her to cook on the stove and stopping her from driving.

These were touchy subjects that she asked about every day. In spite of all the reasons I gave her, she never quit arguing and begging until I told her: "Continuing life without you would be unbearable for me if you died in a house fire or a car accident. I would not be able to forgive myself."

I explained that it wasn't because I thought she was incapable, but simply that her reflexes were delayed and would not allow her enough time to remove herself from danger. Now we don't talk about those areas anymore.

In other areas she is allowed to have quite a bit of control over. But when denying her of privileges that used to be natural for her to do on her own, I relate back to the fact that her children (all of whom do not live in our hometown) entrust me with her safety and well being. And that keeping her safe is my top priority."

- Theresa

"My advice to somebody caring for a Parkinson's sufferer would be:

- Keep them doing normal things, and feeling that they can, for as long as possible.

- Try to stay calm with them, because the mental and physical symptoms will be made worse by stress.

- Have frequent breaks from looking after them: you need somebody else to support you by taking over from time to time. If you get tired and stressed, you won't be much use to the sufferer, so you have to look after yourself as well.

- Put aside part of each day for conversation, as opposed to watching TV or merely dishing out pills and food. Make sure that the conversation involves listening and is two-way.

- In the case of short-term memory loss, it's good to get the sufferer to talk about their past, which they may remember with great clarity, and which will strengthen their sense of identity and worth.

- If the sufferer has a frequent cough, I suggest trying a lactose-free diet, as milk encourages the production of phlegm. There are plenty of good alternatives in food made from soy or rice milk, or vegetable oils."

- Camilla Otaki

"One tip I can pass on is to keep a pencil in your pocket when looking after a Parkinson's sufferer. This is because if they have difficulty mobilizing, the pencil can be placed on the floor in front of them and they will see it as an obstacle and step over it. Once they have got the motion of moving then they will keep going."

- Sharon

"We almost lost my mom because we began attributing every medical problem to her Parkinson's. It turned out that my mom has cancer. My tip? Don't forget to take care of yourself like anyone else."

- Anonymous

"My husband has Parkinson's and dementia. The tip I would give is to get a durable power of attorney (DPOA) early for the spouse (or whomever they wish). I wanted to get the DPOA while my husband still knew what decisions he was making. That way, if my husband has a day where his balance is off or his feet hurt (as he has peripheral neuropathy too) I can take care of business and he doesn't have to feel like he MUST go out or he HAS to do something."

- Mary from Florida, USA

"We use a monitor in my mom's room so my father can hear if she calls out for him because her voice is so weak. He can even go outdoors and still feel as though he is within ear shot. This has given him more freedom."

- Anonymous

"I have learned to have patience and listen to what they have to say. Don't judge them. Let them speak whether it is concerning the subject or not. And please do not rush them. This is my husband's 4th year with Parkinson's. Do not nag them because it confuses them."

- Vera Lewis from Michigan, USA

"If the Parkinson's patient has a hobby, try to encourage it, even if it seems impossible to do or takes hours longer, because it is an outlet. My husband made jewelry but became so discouraged because he said it took two days to do what he used to do in 10 minutes.

I asked him to make something for each of the grandchildren for Christmas. He did and he was busy every day and what joy it was for the grandchildren.

Most people with Parkinson's seem to lose their tempers and especially get angry at the ones they love the most. When that happens, I tell myself this isn't the man I married, it is Parkinson's. It is difficult at times but keep reminding yourself, it helps. That is usually a good time to go to the store and get away for a few minutes so when you come back you can cope once again".

- From a Texas Caregiver

"The only thing that I can mention is that as a wife and a partner who is in love with her husband, I've learned that I should be really supportive and show my love to him every single day and try to encourage him to be strong. I also pray for him and everybody else that has to deal with Parkinson's all the time."

- Anonymous

"The one certain thing that my family has learned is patience. My mom has to be a little bit slower, and take her time at most tasks. Instead of feeling like I need to rush her I take the time to help her any way that I can and treasure every moment that I can spend with her."

- Kathy Vint

"The biggest mistake I have made with my husband who is living with Parkinson's is expecting too much from him. I have to realize that he cannot do things like he use to be able to. He is slower and things are not easy for him to get done.

Things like cooking and chopping vegetables have been difficult. Even though he can still do it, it takes him longer. I need to be patient and give him the freedom to do the task but at his own speed. Patience is the key word in our lives now."

- Linda

"Get ready to be patient as patients are growing slower and slower......expect that. Try to read uplifting articles, TV stories, poems, newspaper clippings of other people adjusting to struggles, cartoons, etc."

- Ann Middleton

"Keep a strong body, mind and soul. Make sure you take time out for yourself, maybe a trip to the gym or a good walk each day, at least 30 minutes. I do this very early before my husband is out of bed in the morning.

We keep a positive approach to the situation, because there is always someone out there worse off than us.

Make the most of the good days and the bad days don't seem quite so hard to take."

- Helen Giltrap from New Zealand

"The number one best advice I think is to get into a support group. You realize that you are not alone, and that goes for both the Parkinsonian and their partner. It's also one of the rare places you can be yourself and not be self-conscious.

We use an egg crate with the top cut off to put all mom's daily pills in. I mark the time with magic marker (7am, 10am, 1pm, 4,pm 7pm, 10pm and B (breakfast) L (lunch) D (dinner) and this way we all know if mom has taken her pills- no second guessing.

Every day is different, every day is special, every day is stressful, BUT I wouldn't trade any of it for the world. My heart has grown 3 sizes.

Be gentle, kind, and loving and of course PATIENT.

What you give, you get back - many times over."

- Mary from Arlington, Virginia, USA

"I purchased a "baby" video monitor to be used when my mother is napping. It is hard for her to talk loud enough to call for help. She also gets confused sometimes when she wakes so remembering to ring the bell we once had isn't working.

Now my Dad can safely do other things in the kitchen and keep watch over her. He can even see when she opens her eyes and is ready for help sitting up.

I bought the one that included two cameras and you can even hear and see in the dark. He appreciates this on those nights when he can't sleep and must get up and be in the other room."

- Leslie Stagner from Lamar, Colorado, USA

"My advice would be to just take each day as it comes and enjoy the blessings around you. My husband continues working each day and I believe that it is the best thing for him now. He is using his vast knowledge about his work and it continues to give him a sense of accomplishment. The people at his office are very supportive and caring.

We continue traveling at every opportunity we can. If there comes a time when we can't, at least we have taken the time now.

I try to provide a stress-free environment for my husband. If something seems too trying, I avoid it, both for him and myself.

Also, LOTS of humor must be interjected. We both laugh off some of the things that he does and I often respond with "I can't believe that you did/said that."

The commitment that we made to each other 43 years ago is really kicking in now. The words, "In Sickness and in Health," are being put to the test. We continue honoring those vows, because I know that if it were me who was undergoing these changes in my life, my husband would be there beside me."

- Judy, Pittsburgh from Pennsylvania, USA

DIAGNOSIS

"Because I have symptoms of bradykinesis, weakness and uncoordination but no tremor, one of the neurologists whom I consulted ordered an MRI. She was the 4th neurologist I consulted.

It showed the ventricles in the brain to be moderately dilated. She believes I may have Normal Pressure Hydrocephalus (NPH) and wants me to have a spinal tap as a diagnostic procedure followed possibly an intraventricular shunt to remove fluid from in and around my brain.

Because I was (am) not eager to have a catheter stuck in my brain I consulted a neurologist at USC for another opinion. He compared the recent MRI with an MRI that was done about 2-3 years ago because I was concerned about memory loss.

Both showed mild to moderate cerebral atrophy consistent with my age and moderate dilatation of the cerebral ventricles. The 2 studies were quite similar.

The USC neurologist does not think I have NPH nor does he think I have Parkinson's. He is planning to discuss it with his colleagues and my Newport Beach neurologist. I have been taking SinemetCR 25-100 about 4 times daily and

I think it helps some.

Summary (so far):

- I don't have a definite diagnosis.
- My walking seems to be about 50% better since I started Sinemet.
- I understand that NPH has symptoms similar to Parkinson's and may respond to Sinemet.
- Most neurologists believe the best treatment is removal of Cerebral Spinal Fluid by means of a shunt in the brain.
- There may be complications associated with intra-cerebral shunts.
- My recent MRI has not changed appreciably for one done about 2 years ago.
- Sinemet seems to help although my walking is certainly not as before.
- I was quite active physically before all this happened but stopped exercising almost completely until I started up again in recent weeks. I don't know which is cause and which is effect.
This is the story so far. I hope this follow up info is helpful. It may be that some other people may have NPH. It is like Parkinson's without the tremor. They may wish to re-evaluate their diagnosis."

- Richard

"I would strongly advise newly diagnosed patients to find a neurologist who has a special interest in PD and is willing to talk openly with you.

I have also noticed situations to avoid are emotional upsets as they worsen your symptoms and sap your energy. If possible try to pace yourself. DO NOT PUSH YOURSELF as PD will kick you back the next day. Have plenty of rest and quiet pastimes.

Try to carry your medication with you at all times and if necessary choose a friendly face to help.

I am concerned about the 'wearing off' factor as it hit me very hard. I wasn't expecting it and wasn't pre-warned. Read all you can about the effectiveness of drugs and their unpredictability. The internet is a wonderful place to find the knowledge to help you and bring you some comfort.

You will feel downhearted from time to time. Unfortunately this is part of the disease. We have to be patient with ourselves and determined to win the fight. Be positive and you will find fulfillment again.

One word frees us of all the weight and pain of life; that word is LOVE."

- Joyce from Winchester, United Kingdom

"Mom hasn't been "officially" diagnosed with PD yet. She has many of the signs and symptoms, as well as many of the difficulties that go along with PD.

She was diagnosed with REM Sleep Behavior Disorder last August. She had been trying to get someone, ANYONE, to listen to her when she told them her stories of horror during sleep. Finally, a pulminologist decided she needed a sleep study. The results were quite frightening! She could not believe she was watching herself on the monitor!

My point is that this particular sleep disorder is said to "cause" PD in some people. It is a disorder normally affecting men, as is Parkinson's. Mom has been struggling with so many of the signs and symptoms of PD for a long time now.

We just weren't aware this is what it was.....or is; and it is so difficult to get a doctor to listen to you sometimes. Especially where we live and especially when my mother has so many health issues. It seems that doctors so often don't know how to "connect the dots".

Mom had a mild stroke in her forties and she has attributed many of her problems to the affects of this. However, we have been learning that with her developing a sleep disorder, she has probably been developing PD all these years as well.

I guess I would just like to make people aware of the possible connection between sleep disorders/behaviors and PD. I am only 43 and a half years old, and am going for my second sleep study in two weeks. I don't have the same disorder as my mother; but a problem nonetheless.

It is said that PD is not "hereditary". However, I believe that families can have the same predisposition. My husband's grandmother has three siblings with PD. One of them has already passed away."

- Sandy McCoy from St. Francois County, Missouri, USA

"I have found out that I have been flagged as a patient of PSP (Progressive Supra Nuclear Palsy) which has many similarities to Parkinson's.

It is certainly nice to know what disease one has. The really big item in my life these days is my wife, Sandie. She has taken control over many things that have affected my well being, and works on them daily with me. Something like getting up from a chair properly so you do not fall over backwards (as I was doing from time to time) is one of the big problems with PSP.

As a matter of fact Sandie has been so attentive to me and my problems associated to PSP that my neurologist is extremely impressed with my stability, or as I sometimes see it, "my progress".

I think PSP is something that perhaps all patients of Parkinson's (or their caregivers) should know about as it is a relatively new disease. It may turn out that instead of suffering from Parkinson's, the patient may really be a victim of PSP."

- Clancy MacDonald from North Bay, Ontario, Canada

DOCTORS

"A woman whose husband had Parkinson's told me soon after my husband was diagnosed nearly 14 years ago, "How your husband does will depend completely on who your doctor is." She was right, and I would go a step further: "How your husband does, AND HOW YOU DO will depend completely on who your doctor or doctors are."

A team of top-notch doctors who embrace both traditional and alternative medicines and treatments, who collaborate with each other and with me, have made a tremendous difference in our quality of life.

If your doctor doesn't suggest it, help yourself out by looking into the many alternative treatments that are available today. And, by all means, join the Well Spouse Association. Their newsletter Mainstay can be a lifesaver for the spousal caregiver."

- Amie from New York, USA

"It is important to remember that the doctor is not God. If something doesn't work right or doesn't feel right for you, get a second opinion. Jim's doctor had him on 27 mg of Requip per day.

We finally went to another doctor for a re-evaluation and they completely took him off of all the Requip. He not only feels better, the hallucinations have stopped. He is no longer a "space cadet", falling asleep everywhere."

- Jim and Nola from New Port Richey, Florida, USA

DRESSING

"I had a hip replaced in 1992 and was given what I call a grabber and a sock aid which I still use. The grabber is about two feet long and enables me to pick things up without bending over. The sock aid is a piece of plastic with a puller string attached. You thread the sock on the plastic to pull your sock on."

- Jim Ferguson

DROOLING

"His excessive drooling is being controlled with this new doctor putting him on Artane. That has really been good for his self-esteem. The drooling was very unsettling to him. The first doctor had him on Artane also but with everything else he was taking, it was just too much for his system."

- Jim and Nola from New Port Richey, Florida, USA

"For all PD patients, drooling is a quality of life issue. For some, drooling becomes so bad that it prevents them from socializing because they don't want to be seen in public constantly drooling. This was the case for my father. He couldn't use any of the anticholinergic drugs (such as Artane) because he had a propensity to hallucinations and these type of drugs tended to exacerbate these symptoms. Speech therapy exercises were not helpful either. You see, constant drooling has nothing to do with increased saliva output but is caused by reduced frequency in swallowing. This is why a speech therapist is used – to try and teach the patient to swallow more often. Unfortunately, for my father, this did not work.

On October 1, 2006, the Centers for Medicare and Medicaid approved payment for the use of injections of Botulinum Toxin Type A (Botox) to help reduce drooling (also called sialorrhea). Of course, health care professionals have to provide the proper documentation to support the use of these injections but I feel it is important to know that there is another alternative out there for patients who have not been relieved of their problem of massive drooling by any other means.

Your health care provider should know the proper coding for the use of these injections but after careful research, I found when reporting an injection of Botulinum Toxin Type A the following pairing of CPT codes and ICD-9-CM codes should be used:

CPT: 42699 (injection salivary glands)
ICD-9-CM: 527.7 - Disturbance of salivary secretion

If you share this information with your health care provider, you will finally find some relief."

- Jean Moffat

DRY MOUTH

"I had a major problem with an extremely dry mouth while sleeping at night (possibly due to the Mirapex I take before bedtime). My doctor recommended rinsing my mouth with Biotene Mouthwash (a "Mouthwash for Dry Mouth Care") before going to bed, and it really made a difference. It is available at any drug store and has a very pleasant taste."

- Anonymous

EATING

"My mother had difficulty getting the utensils into her mouth so I purchased utensils that you can bend in whatever direction to make it easier to eat. My father was amazed how much quicker my mother was able to finish her meal. The soup spoon was especially helpful. Maybe my mother will even gain some weight now!"

- Anonymous

"My wife carries a small top quality vegetable paring knife (Victorinox brand) with her when going out for a meal. This is because her right arm is the weak one and so it helps in cutting up her food. Now she doesn't always have to resort to me."

- Chris Tuttle

"I'm still trying to find the right dosage of medicine to (hopefully) stop the tremors in my hands.

I did come upon a neat trick to help with the shakes when I am trying to eat dinner. The tremors seem to be stronger in my right hand which happens to be the hand I use the most.

When I get ready to eat dinner I place my left and on my lap and deliberately start shaking my left hand. The shaking in my right hand stops long enough for me to eat several forks full of food.

I'm not sure how long this little "trick" will work but it has made eating easier for the last couple of weeks. Now if I could only find a "trick" that would help me drink my glass of milk......other than using a straw."

- Yvonne from Maryland, USA

EXERCISE

"I have some advice: EXERCISE, EXERCISE, EXERCISE! Try to walk 20 minutes every day, do 15 to 20 minutes of floor exercises every day, as well as stretching, and use 1 pound weights.

It is enormously important and helpful to start this as soon as one is diagnosed with PD. It does wonders for walking and balance issues."

- Shirlee from Alabama, USA

"No matter how bad your symptoms are, keep moving as much as possible. I have been on a physical therapy program for the past 3 months and it has made a significant difference in my ability to function."

- Anonymous

"I can only think of Pilates. I take a private Pilates lesson once a week on the machines, and it helps so much.

I asked our former governor who also has PD (l5 years) and just had successful DBS surgery and he said, exercise, exercise, exercise!

There are glutathione patches available now but I just started using it today. I am going to try gene therapy (Google gene therapy for Parkinson's). I use the internet A LOT!"

- Mary Ellen

"What I do know works for me is getting out and doing something active. Yesterday I went horse riding with my daughter. I hadn't been out riding for a year, and it was brilliant. The horse gives you your legs and balance and I felt 'normal' trotting and cantering along the country lanes on a beautiful, cold but sunny February day!

Last week I went for a swim, and again, swimming is easy – it's the walking that's hard for us!

Exercise is important for everybody, but for me with PD it lifts body, mind and soul - you can actually forget about having PD (now wouldn't that be nice)."

- Aideen

"Up to this point with my Parkinson's disease, I'd say that exercise is my answer to help me deal with it. I obtained an exercise notebook and DVD from the Parkinson's Disease Foundation and it has been a tremendous help. It is filled with exercises which are great and easy to do, plus I do a few Yoga stretching positions every day.

I also go to the YMCA and use the treadmill for walking, the stationary bike and various weight equipment three times a week.

Walking is difficult, but can be done by taking big steps at a rapid rate. Remember to walk, heel down first and up on your toes."

- Pat Quinn from Waxhaw, North Carolina, USA

"The thing that I have discovered that has had the greatest positive impact on my daily life with Parkinson's is good old EXERCISE. You don't have to set up an Olympic training camp. I'm talking about two 30 to 40 minute programs that you can alternate depending on the weather.

Walking is great as well as Yoga and Pilates - anything that helps keep your joints moving.

Shortly after I was diagnosed I went to a fitness trainer and she set me up with a program that is simple and quite rewarding and I added a few of my own. You would be surprised at how many trainers work with Parkinson's patients.

That's it, simple and effective. My neurologist at my last visit told me that if he didn't know better he wouldn't be able to diagnose me with Parkinson's."

- Gerard

"This works pretty good for me. I am a golf professional and caddie which keeps me active. I walk and run between 5-10 miles a day on the golf course.

I take 2 Aleve arthritis pills a day which allows my joints to move a lot freer, a multivitamin, and three Carbidopa and 2 Selegiline pills a day. The Carbidopa allows my body to function better and it lasts about 5 hours for me. I don't take any more Carbidopa than I have to because I don't like the jittery after affects.

I lift weights 5 days a week and use free weights to keep my strength and balance up. I have found that lifting weights relaxes my muscles and gives me better muscle control. I will admit that at times my joints were very painful and it took a lot of mental toughness to keep lifting through it but I did and I still play golf and still score in the 70's.

Hopefully this will help someone else. I just refuse to let this take me over and I will keep fighting it as long as I can and as long as I am able to."

- Mike

"Physical therapy and exercise have helped very much, especially exercising in the pool. Unloading the dishwasher helps him too. It takes him awhile but it does get him to reach up into the cupboards to put things away and he tries to make a point of doing that every day.

He feels that the stretching is good for him."

- Jim and Nola from New Port Richey, Florida, USA

"I probably have early stage Parkinson's but it has been with me at least four years. I've found that I can control my left hand trembling and foot "cogging" by doing isometric exercises with my hands and feet twice a day.

I stretch the palms of my hands as hard as I can for 20 seconds, three times and then do the same with my feet. With the hands, after each stretch, I rapidly open and close them into a fist ten times. With the feet, after each stretch, I slowly and smoothly push the feet down flat to the floor."

- Norm from Florida, USA

"My wife really finds relief in her weekly massage and has also completed a Pilate's course specifically aimed at improving balance and lengthening tendons, muscles, etc. to counteract the early indications."

- Chris Tuttle

"I find the most important thing I can do is aerobic exercise. I do a minimum of 20 minutes a day 5-6 days a week. Generally 30 minutes is best.

I find that it forces my body to produce dopamine and that for brief periods of time I feel the way I did before the disease.

I also do weight bearing exercises to strengthen the muscles on my left side which is weaker than my right. When I am at work I keep a stress ball in my left hand and squeeze it to help maintain the dexterity and strength in that hand."

- Barbara

"I schedule exercise into my life instead of exercising when it's convenient. I've read that exercise can allow a person to reduce the dosage of medicine by half. So exercising and not focusing on PD is the most helpful to me and it allows me to live life normally."

- Anonymous

"My best advice is exercise, exercise, exercise! Just 10-15 minutes a day makes a big difference in handling stress, physical abilities and just feeling good."

- Darlene Calabrese

"I exercise - my brain by writing poetry, my hands by practising writing, my face muscles by smiling!"

- Lindsey Priest from Hornsea, England

"My best advice is to never stop exercising, even if it is difficult. I am also a firm believer that prayer changes things."

- Terry

"Encourage playing 18 holes of golf two to three times a week. Sure they are slow putting the tee down, positioning the ball, whatever...just take a separate cart from the group and tell them you don't want to slow them down. Also keep the tees snug under the side of your cap for easy retrieval."

- Diana Rowlett from Texas, USA

"I found if my husband stays very active he does better both physically and mentally. So I suggest not sitting around feeling sorry for oneself."

- Anonymous

"One thing I think is very important to do is to exercise. I go to the fitness center 3 times a week. Aside from being enjoyable, the benefits are many. I believe it keeps me flexible, at least more flexible than I would be if I didn't go."

- Barbara

"I was diagnosed with PD January of 2005 at age 56. My symptoms are slight - I am still in the first stage. I was always very active and when diagnosed I decided that I would continue doing everything that I was already doing as long as I possibly could.

I went to physical therapy to see what sort of exercises would help to keep me limber and incorporated them into the exercises that I was already doing. It is my hope that staying active will help me to delay some of the effects of the disease.

Obviously it is much too soon to determine success or failure but at least I feel like I am doing something positive. Check back with me in a few years and I will let you know how I am making out.

Meanwhile here is a list of some of the things I do: several stretches every morning, 50 push ups and 100 sit-ups 3 mornings a week, walking and running - combined total of over 1000 miles each of the last 2 years (and 14 years prior to being diagnosed).

I also ran a 5k race and a 4.5 mile race this past year finishing in the top half both overall and in my age group, rock climbing at a local gym 1-2 times a week and outdoor climbing (lead, sport and top rope) several times a year, occasional bike riding and hiking. Again, it is too early to say if all of this will help physically (especially in the long haul) but it certainly helps my mental outlook now.

- Lee Lamison

"See a physical therapist that specializes in Parkinson's, specifically gait and posture. The earlier you do this the better but it is never too late.

Become "addicted" to the exercise/stretching routines you are given. Do them daily (spread them out over the day if that helps) for 6 weeks and you will know what I mean by "addicted".

Get feedback on your progress by observing your gait and posture in a mirror or reflective window or have a friend take a video of you walking. A bent forward shuffle feels normal after a while if we don't work on gait and posture and it causes a series of stresses on our bodies that we don't want or need.

Here is one exercise to get started: While sitting on the edge of your bed, or forward in a chair, round your lower spine as far back as you can and hold for 3 seconds. Then curve it forward as far as you can for 3 seconds. Think of moving your belly button backward and forward. Focus on your lower back and let your shoulders hang normally. Work up to 10 repetitions and do this twice a day.

Your correct posture should be with your belly button forward and that probably is not normal for you now, is it? With your lower spine curved back notice the stress in your neck because your head is bent forward. With your lower spine curved forward (belly button forward) notice how your whole spine straightens and the muscles in your neck can relax because they aren't having to keep your head, which is almost as heavy as a bowling ball, from falling forward.

Over the course of a day you will relieve considerable stress by sitting and standing with the belly button forward posture. With two minutes work a day this posture will soon feel normal to you and your neck and back will thank you."

- Bruce Higgins from Gig Harbor, Washington, USA

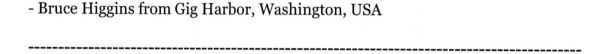

"I find that I am controlling the disease well due to yoga exercise. Every morning before breakfast, I walk 1 to 2 miles a day, still golf once a week and bowl with the 10 pins. I have a positive attitude and face every day with courage and determination."

- Simone Valade from Ontario, Canada

"I was diagnosed in the late 90's at the ripe old age of 48 or there abouts. Although I noticed things a couple of years before that, and felt that there was something just not right. I am usually a pretty good judge when things seem to be going wrong or whatever.

My journey thus far fighting this disease has been a lot of education, a lot of reading and teaching myself how to deal with it. As you know it affects everyone differently.

One thing I know for sure is that we need to keep moving as much as we possibly can. Exercise, exercise, exercise. I play tennis which really keeps me moving, not competitively anymore but for the social aspect and the enjoyment of the game. It is GREAT.

I also believe that we must keep it together as much as possible. We must PUSH ourselves. My husband says I'm a bullhead because I never ask for help when I'm doing things as they can take me longer to do, and it can be frustrating to all concerned.

I lift weights; 5lbs. and 10lbs. on a good day. I try to walk every day which really feels good for the mind as well as getting the fresh air for your body as well. It gets the endorphins working and you just plain feel better.

I still work 3-4 days a week too. The disease tries to get to you but I cannot stress it enough that exercise really is a must and very beneficial to keeping the mind focused and you do not need an attitude adjustment as often.

Yes, there are days of grey and depression tries to get you, but pull yourself together and go for a walk and that will get you back to square one..

So I guess to sum it all up the most important thing in my mind is exercise so if that helps anyone fighting this disease okay, I have contributed something.

I truly do believe EXERCISE is the number one key to slowing this very progressive disease."

- Judy Johnson from Stanwood, Washington, USA

MEDICATION

"I think that everyone should know about the possible side effects of higher doses of Mirapex. My husband had been online gambling for nearly 10 months to a year before I found out. We lost over $160,000 to gambling.

The connection was the amount of Mirapex he was taking. When the doctor lowered the dosage, the desire went away for my husband. He had no prior interest in gambling until the doses increased. I hope this will help others before it is too late."

- Lisa

"I was diagnosed with PD in 2005. For the past 2 years I have been experimenting with new drugs but I have had some unpleasant side effects with drugs like Amantadine and Rasagiline.

I have finally come to terms with Sinemet 25/100 and Zelapar (the melting tab on the tongue). I take 2-1-2 of Sinemet and 1 of Zelapar. It seems to work well for my PD. Even my doctor remarked that I am doing well."

- Sarala

"At the time of this writing, my husband is on an experimental drug sponsored by Novartis and supplied by his neurologist. One pill three times a day and NO side effects.

Let me tell you, what a difference this has made in his life, to the point where he has been able to go back to work full time. This is a 9 month study and we have even discovered a way to stay on the medication after the study is over for no charge to us.

This is already available in the US, but won't be available in Canada until at least 2008 or later. This is one drug that should be available sooner and the tab should be picked up by the government."

- Julie Berger

"I was in a pilot program for a new drug, or fairly new from Israel called Azilect. This program was with a doctor from Dallas, Texas named Dr. Malcolm Stewart. He is a doctor that sees strictly Parkinson's patients.

There were 10 of us living in the metroplex at that time on this particular program. This drug is supposed to help keep Parkinson's from progressing as fast as it would otherwise.

I am in early stages, so not sure about it yet. I am now on a smaller dose of Azilect, along with Benzatropine. I feel that it helps with the tremor most of the time, which is the only symptom I have as of now. Occasionally I shake in my left leg or foot.

Ultimately it would be wonderful if they could come up with a pill that just stops the problem in its path. I am sure we all feel this way of course........Maybe in time they will?"

- Sue

"I am a dentist who works full time teaching at Nova Southeastern University and I spent more than year learning to utilize my Sinemet prescription so that it would work throughout the day while I was teaching at school.

I found that using a "timer" to insure taking my medication on time would be the only way to consistently reap the benefits that the Sinemet can provide. I would also like to advise my fellow sufferers to be careful when introducing a new medication and even drugs that behave or deliver Sinemet like pharmaceuticals because they potentially can cause undesirable side affects especially over the long run.

I personally had a problem with Stelevo which played havoc with my system for several months until my neurologist figured it out. We eliminated that drug from my useful list."

-Norman Feigenbaum

"This advice is for the newly diagnosed. One doctor told me that it is not good to over medicate. He says treat the symptoms you can't live with and live with the symptoms you can endure. Over medication can bring serious side effects (painful constipation, heavy drowsiness during the day, serious back pain, rapid blinking, etc.).

I followed this advice and removed one medication from my regimen. I feel a lot better and more importantly, can function satisfactorily."

- Anonymous

"I know since my husband has been on the new drug Azilect, I have seen a remarkable improvement in his self-confidence. He now will go to the mall and walk on his own, he will now drive more often and he also does a two mile walk down the beach. He just seems to have a lot more energy and better outlook. Hope this helps anyone who is thinking of trying this drug."

- Ann Furey

"I find that if my husband takes his meds in the middle of the night it helps him to get up in the morning. He takes Sinemet 4 times a day (every 4 hours) and the last one is at 8 PM. So if he takes one when he wakes up through the night he can get up better in the morning."

- Patricia

"I have found out from the Support Nurse of my local branch that antibiotics are a big no no if you take Sinemet. It cancels out the medication so beware being prescribed antibiotics for whatever reason."

- Drew

"Mom was diagnosed with Parkinson's Dementia about 1 and a half years ago. She was put on Aricept which turned her around 100% for about a week. We then began seeing some of the same forgetfulness and confusion again.

We were able to deal with everything until about two months ago when my brother who lives above Mom and oversees her daily care went back to work fulltime. Our main issue was her meds.

We had four cases clearly marked 10:00, 3:00, 8:00 and bedtime, Monday-Friday and an Atomic clock showing the day of the week. One Tuesday my brother came home from work about 5:00 to discover that Mom had taken T-W-TH-F-S 3:00 meds all in one day.

I thought the time had come to discuss a nursing home with her. Instead I turned to the internet where I previously saw very expensive medication dispensers. I was hoping to find a more reasonable, easy to operate dispenser with 4 daily med times.

I found one with 28 pill slots, ordered it and took it to Mom's as soon as it arrived. My brother and I spent about 1 hour programming, and filling the dispenser. It is great. It is about the size of a dinner plate and, it has a lock so Mom can only get to the one dose available.

She no longer has the anxiety connected with trying to remember to take her meds, because an alarm sounds at the dosage time. And she doesn't have to match the day on the clock to the day on the proper med case. All she has to do is slide the door open, take her meds out, and slide the door shut. It has made dealing with Mom and her meds a breeze.

I recommend this MedRedi dispenser. I paid $150 total for the device which includes a dispenser tray and an extra dispenser tray. I highly recommend this item for any caregivers who are experiencing this type of problem."

- Debbie Filling

"I found another drug from Israel. I asked my doctor about it, and he said that if I could get it, take it. It was NOT okayed here in the States until 2006. But I got it through IsraMeds which is a discount pharmacy in Israel.

It is called Azilect (Rasagiline). I started taking it in May of 2005. After about 3 months, I noticed that I was snapping my fingers on my left hand while listening to the radio in my car. I was having much difficulty with that hand. I feel that it is holding me at where I was at that time. I have stayed just about the same. Unless I do not get much sleep, then I notice a slight difference.

Anyone can get this from Israel. They are at www.IsraMeds.com and you can phone direct 866-477-2289 or 877-471-7247 and their email is Order@IsraMeds.com. I usually speak with Ron. They also phone every few months to see how you are doing.

I take one every morning with breakfast. I do not know what the cost is here now, in America, but I do think it is less in Israel. I know the price dropped in Israel when it became available here. Hope this helps anyone who can take this pill."

- Jaynie B. Kane

"Here is something I have found helpful for my dad. Being that both my parents take many medicines, my mom is the one who has had to try to keep track of what and when my dad should take his meds.

His Parkinson's has caused him to not remember when or if he took his medicines so I decided to buy a timer for him to set after taking his first dose of the day (he takes his meds 4 times a day every 4 hours).

Additionally, we keep a pad and pen next to timer so when the timer goes off, he takes his meds, writes down the time he took them and resets the timer. This has really been a great help for both my parents, allowing my dad to be independent even though he gets a little reminder for the timer!"

- Sherri Pensler from Miami, Florida, USA

"My wife Janice was diagnosed with Parkinson's about four years ago.

The most significant improvement in her condition came about when she was given a new drug, Razadyne ER a year ago. It is a form of Galantamine. It is more commonly prescribed for Alzheimer's, which her neurologist assures us she does not have.

The biggest improvement has been in her energy level, her morale, and her cognitive abilities. She still has the same tremors which were not affected.

The Razadyne is in addition to all the other drugs commonly prescribed for Parkinson's. "

- Anonymous

"I was diagnosed with PD 19 months ago. My doctor immediately put me on Levodopa and then about six months later he added Requip (.5mg 3xday).

While the Levodopa restored my motion, I was bothered by stiffness (especially in my left arm). Then after 9 months or so, I was experiencing frequent facial muscle contractions and twitching. After 15 months I noticed that after any strenuous activity (like yard work or moving a heavy object) I was left exhausted with internal body trembling.

Two months ago I read about a medication called Azilect. I have been on Azilect (.5mg 1xday) for about 6 weeks now. I had heard it may cause heartburn type problems so I take the one pill in the morning with food.

I noticed marked improvement after the week or so. I feel almost normal again. The stiffness has subsided noticeably and I have more strength to do the physical activities that were not possible before. The only side effect was some constipation which went away after 3-4 weeks.

I am amazed, grateful, and hopeful the positive effects will continue longer term."

- Anonymous

"I would like to mention a certain thing about allergic reaction to Carbadopa/Levodopa. Shortly after starting this medication, my Dad broke out in a rash. Over a 6 month period we eliminated all medications except for Carb/Levo and he still had the rash. This was a scratch until you bleed rash!

Through luck, we determined that the Carbadopa was causing the rash. Levodopa (by itself) has not been manufactured since March 2005. I had Levodopa compounded and the rash went away. You can take Levodopa for only so long before its effectiveness runs out (apparently).

A different neurologist recommended Comtan to be taken with the Levodopa and said that Comtan works pretty much the same as Carbadopa. My first thought ... if it works the same as Carbadopa will it produce the same rash?!

This time I asked for a sample of the medication. (Sam's Club priced the medication at $361.00 for a 30 day supply.) After taking the medication for about three days, here comes the scratching and after 5 days, it is the same old RASH! At least I don't have 25 days of this medication sitting with 25 days of several other medications! (I do have some Carbadopa/Levodopa 25/100 and 25/250)."

- Rich

MIND

"The only tip I have is to keep your body and mind busy. Do some writing and some reading every day. Write a story, or start writing your memoirs. I finished mine and gave copies to my children and grandchildren. Try writing some poetry or a short fictional story."

- Harlan

"For me personally retaining my sense of humor is vital. It is so important to see the funny side of life. It is so easy to slip into a depressive state especially when the tremors get bad and one goes "off". Seek out people who make you laugh. After all life is not a rehearsal - what we have is IT so make the best of IT."

- Drew

MOBILITY/GETTING AROUND

"One suggestion I might make is if you're on a walker and you stand up after sitting for a while, be sure to get your balance before beginning to walk. He didn't and he fell, hitting the hearth of the fireplace and bursting his one and only kidney."

- LaVeta

"I have been freezing going into doors for 5 years now and holding everyone up behind me (really embarrassing). This was first due to my having Parkinson's and now also due to a very bad fall I had last November (fractured my pelvis in two places).

I had to have a lot of therapy and the therapist I had also helped me with my PD. She told me to take longer steps when I walk and don't tell your brain to do anything (I used to say "STEP OVER" when I would get to a door). Well I did what she told me to do and low and behold it worked!

I have never felt so good. It feels so natural now to walk. I still have a problem with turning around and my balance (which was why I fell down) but I am working on it.

I also take CoQ10 200mg a day which my PD doctor recommended and I feel I have more energy. I have to tell you he could not believe it when I walked into his office without freezing at his door! What a beautiful thing."

- Moe

"Bob and I have found that using bottom satin sheets and satin underwear makes it a whole lot easier to be able to turn over in the bed. I still have to help him but cotton shorts don't slide very well.

You may have already discovered this as well. With his drooling I purchased some western like bandanas and I tie these around his neck as the cowboys do and this keeps his undershirt and shirt dry. I hope this us useful for someone."

- Joanne

"One of the difficulties with Parkinson's patient of course is their mobility. Sometimes getting a patient in and out of bed or the car can be challenging.

For the car I had the passenger seat moved back about two inches because Mom was having trouble bending her legs enough to clear the door jam. This was a great help but she still had problems scooting herself back into the seat and turning her body to face forward.

I now place a plastic bag down on the seat before she sits down which makes it easier for her to move or for me to help adjust her. This worked so well in the car that I decided to try it in her bed.

I have always used a bed pad or sheet under her to help slide her up or down but this was difficult also. I placed the garbage bag under the mattress pad and now when I turn her from a sitting position to a lying down position it is so easy for both of us. I can also pull her up and down in bed by myself now also."

- Kay

"A fine walking aid that my husband discovered is the use of our grandson's (outgrown) baby buggy (rubber-wheeled stroller) as his walker. It absorbs pavement bumps, is more stable than the usual walker, has brakes and carrying space, and elicits friendly comments from other pedestrians. ("What a cute baby!")

I have added an 8 lb. weight for increased stability. He now feels safer, more comfortable and carefree as he strolls around the neighborhood."

- Alice from El Cerrito, California, USA

"When I feel my muscles going into the 'shut-down' mode, I try to rest! If I catch the episodes early enough, the pain is less and I am able to recover faster."

- Anonymous

"It is important to remember to get rid of the throw rugs. I thought they would be okay since they all had rubber backing but they weren't. Our floor is tile and he has finally learned to slow down and pivot when he turns around. He constantly has to remind himself to not hurry and not keep his feet too close together when he walks."

- Jim and Nola from New Port Richey, Florida, USA

"My tip concerns walking which is often difficult for me after 14 years with Parkinson's.

I get started most easily if I imagine big, colored footprints leading forward from me, and then proceed to step on the footprints. It gets me going. Once I get going, I try to find my "natural" pace--one that is in tune with the frequency of a pendulum representing my body while walking. This pace I try to maintain so that I don't regress into a shuffle.

For me, this "natural" pace is fairly brisk, like 3-4 mph. The imagining of footsteps is also useful when maneuvering to sit in a chair or negotiate through a crowd of people."

- Rob Fish from Aptos, California, USA

"One of the pitfalls of PD is that one tends to lose balance more often and we have to guard against this. Never be too proud to use a cane or a walker when you become aware of your need for such assistance.
I speak from experience here because on December 23rd I fell in my home and broke my hip, which necessitated replacement surgery on Christmas day and a 3

week stay in the hospital. I am home again and recovering with physiotherapy, and the help of a walker and also a cane. (Previously I was using a cane only)."

- Nancy Fox

"I advise getting grab rails at strategic points when your balance is as poor as mine is. About three years ago, I read somewhere that satin sheets would assist in turning in bed. I happened to mention this to my morning caregiver and asked if any of her clients had them. She quickly replied "Yes, and don't worry, they are not kinky."

I got the sheets which have been a success and at the time wrote this little poem:

These satin sheets are nice and slinky,
though some folk think they are rather kinky.
But now I'm nearing seventy seven,
and no longer expect a Seventh Heaven.
These sheets, alas it must be said,
are only to help me turn over in bed."

- Arthur from England

"Another helpful item is using gripper socks to get more traction under foot when getting out of bed."

- Anonymous

"I've had a shaking hand for 2 years and my doctor insists it's Parkinson's. It quite often shakes while playing games on the computer but I've found that putting an Ace bandage on the wrist has stopped the shaking and has stopped a lot of unwanted extra clicks."

-Roger from Hamburg, New York, USA

"My husband was diagnosed with Parkinson's disease 7 years ago. He has had walking problems, a strange gait, and pitches forward all the time so he falls over very easily.

He has been going to exercise classes and the physiotherapist has provided him with a very long pole with a rubber stopper on the end. This has enabled him to walk more comfortably and in a more upright position. There is also less jolting when he walks and he is more stable, thus reducing the chance of experiencing falls.

We have been able to take up walking again, which in the past was his favorite hobby (we used to walk from 8 to 12 miles in a day). He is now able to do up to 3 miles at a time and we are hoping to gradually increase it."

- Eileen Bailey from Shrewsbury, England

"Use satin or silk sheets or pajamas - it's so much easier to turn over in bed."

- Beth from Australia

"I have a tremor in my left arm, and am left handed. I have found that if I knit or occupy my hand with something the tremors stop. I send my knitted things to charity places which also makes me feel there is something worthwhile in this disease."

- Anonymous

"I am in the early stages of Parkinson's and have a hard time when my hand shakes. I have learned that my dominant hand shakes at rest, and when my hand and arm begins to ache, I know the shaking is about to begin. It doesn't always happen when it's almost time for medication.

I embroider, work on a quilt, or play with a rubber ball, lightly squeezing and releasing it. Anything to keep my hand busy to lessen the shaking, or stop it entirely. I am fortunate to have wonderful friends and a thoughtful husband who does anything to help me."

- Anonymous

"When I am at the end of my walking time and I am stuck, I get behind one of my friends or family members and ask them to walk ahead of me so I can watch them. Then I follow their foot steps. Sometimes they can walk ahead, or if I am really tired they walk backwards and I look down at their feet. It seems like I have to learn to walk all over again, but it works for me.

Also, when I am at a party and there is music, I am able to get up with the grandchildren and dance. Not for a long evening, but for a few songs. I am not a dancer and can't carry a tune, but music keeps me going.
I have had PD for 24 years. I am 78 years old and on medication every 4 hours, 24 hrs a day. I try to keep up driving as long as I feel I am not endangering any one, and I try to keep a positive outlook. I will go until I drop and refuse to give up.

I keep up with the news and follow a sport; I follow the COLTS. I keep up with the grandkids by email, read, and go out for dinner. My hobby is art and I keep my mind busy.

I never give up and thank the Lord I am even able to share this with others."

- Jean Boring

"My tip for anyone who has PD and has lost the dexterity in their fingers is to learn to play the piano or organ and play it at least twice daily.

It is such a wonderful hobby even if you can't carry a tune but can learn to make music by reading notes."

- Anonymous

"The one thing that seems to happen sometimes with my Mum is a feeling of light-headedness, usually when standing up. I believe it's to do with low blood pressure caused by PD. It might seem obvious, but I don't think PD sufferers should try and move until this feeling is past, because it could cause them to fall"

- Anonymous

NAUSEA

"Like many other people on this type of medication, I have suffered from nausea as a result of taking these pills. However, by complete accident, I discovered that I felt less nauseous when we were away on holidays and traveling around in the car.

170

When I evaluated the situation, the only difference I could find was that I was wearing travel bands (for travel sickness). These are called 'Sea Bands' in this country and look like grey elastic bracelets.

They are said to work by acting on the acupuncture points on the inside of the wrists. Whatever they did, they seemed to work for me, so I hope that someone else might be able to benefit from them too."

- Margaret from United Kingdom

NUTRITION AND SUPPLEMENTS

"My sister has Parkinson's and her most difficult obstacle has been lack of energy.

Luckily, my pastor's wife told me about a vitamin mineral supplement called "Reliv". I began taking the product myself and found it increased my energy level dramatically. I sent some to my sister and she is thrilled with the results!! I can tell a difference just in the strength of her voice (we live in different cities)."

- Anonymous

"My mother is real close to stage 5 of P.D. and not interested in eating anything other than waffles with syrup and fruit, three times a day, seven days a week. We were having a difficult time with this due to the obvious, not enough balanced nutrition.

Mom would communicate that every time she would think of putting anything else in her mouth she would get nauseous. We would still keep trying to get her to eat a variety of foods. The result would be that she didn't eat much.
It wasn't until I bought a brand of waffles that she wasn't used to eating that I realized just how sensitive her taste buds were! Mom couldn't eat the new brand.

So, now we realize this was a real thing, and we would rather have Mom eating well and enough to keep her strength up as well as enjoying her meals. She does take a multivitamin as hard as it is to swallow them.

I hope someone else who might be going though this with their loved one can take comfort in knowing it is okay to let go of some things."

- Shirley from Maine, USA

"After several months of taking Requip my husband was like a zombie all hunched over with his arms dragging. His daughter was in Oregon teaching yoga and came home with a bottle of StemEnhance. He told her he would take it to see if it would do him any good.

He took two a day and in four days he was walking upright. He no longer shuffles unless he is very tired. We went to his neurologist and were told if it does you this much good, go for it. He hasn't had any worse tremors and his salivating has lessened considerably.

What it does is it promotes the person's adult stem cells into helping with the part that is damaged. I recommend it highly. One member of the PD group of Memphis started taking it and no longer has to use a walker and takes fewer shots for pain. She is 38 and it has done her a great deal of good. It is a capsule of green algae. You can look it up on the internet at Stem Tech.com."

- Anonymous

"The only special thing I am doing is 1200mg of Coenzyme Q10 every day as per a study that determined that it slows the progression of the disease."

- Marv Siegal

"Recently my wife read on the net that blueberries / blueberry juice was good for Parkinson's so I have been having a 6 oz glass of juice a day for about 3 weeks now.

My wife said she has noticed a difference at nighttime as I don't seem to dream as much and I am more relaxed."

- Donat Bouchard from 100 Mile House, British Columbia, Canada
"Most brain diseases are a result of lack of oxygen. One of the primary causes is probably arthrosclerosis (hardening of the arteries).

The medical profession believes that most adults in the western world have this disease that seriously affects blood flow throughout the body, including the brain. Blood is the primary (only) source of oxygen to the brain cells. When your doctor discovers blockage in the carotid arteries, there is no doubt blockage throughout the other 25 thousand miles of veins, etc. in your body, including the brain.

There is strong opinion throughout many segments of the scientific and medical communities that a change in diet is REQUIRED. Fruits, vegetables, omega 3

172

fats, whole grains (ex. no Trans fats, no red meats).

This approach won't work overnight, considering that it took many years of wrong diet to create the problem. Many professionals believe that good blood flow to the brain cells will eventually correct these brain deficiencies.

I am a retired engineer, with no training in the medical field. The above info is my opinion, based on all of my reading of the literature over the past three years."

 - Tom

"My Mom was toxic to fast foods and poor nutrition, not eating fresh fruits and vegetables. Adding more water to her diet daily has helped her have BM's daily and has helped her movement.

She also started Coenzyme Q10, 1200 mg through Life Extension. This is a lot cheaper than anywhere else and it is of good quality. She also takes a good vitamin supplement through The Vitamin Shoppe.

Prayer and thankfulness to God who keeps her well daily is important. In a nutshell, this has delayed her symptoms and keeps her functional. A massage and acupuncture from time to time also helps her."

 - Amber Foguth

PAIN

"About 14 months ago I developed pain in my lower spine area and had cramps shooting down my right leg. It was very similar to a sciatica attack. I have been seen by three specialists, sent for x-rays and CT scans yet no one knows for sure what is causing this.

I went for acupuncture but did not feel that it did anything for me. I took prescription pain killers which also did not help. I still have this pain which now comes on in the late evenings. Since the onset of this problem I cannot sit for long or stand for long or walk for long!

The most acceptable explanation came from the specialist treating me for my Parkinsonian syndrome. He felt that this pain was due to my being on Bromocriptine for too long (approx 6 years). He changed the prescription and now I take Mirapex 1 mg tabs 3 times a day. I still continue to take Sinemet CR 100/25 1 tab 4 times per day.

I have found massage therapy extremely helpful. I have 2 hours of therapy twice a week and my RMT who is very good has been able to get this awful pain to a manageable level."

- Jacine

"I have found a device called Medicure quite effective for pain relief in my back which is my principle problem. It is absolutely marvelous for the relief of muscle cramps which I am afflicted with especially in bed when exercising.

The most effective setting for me for cramp relief is 20Hz. The device which is made in the UK by Snowden Healthcare Ltd in Nottingham works through Natural Magnetic Field Therapy."

- David

"I have a tip for you and it is about a massager I had bought for massaging a painful knee. About a year and half ago I was having a terrible problem with one knee and saw this massager on TV called "DR-HO'S Massage System" (www.drhonow.com) and thought it just might help me. In 10 days I was walking with no pain."

- Maurice DeWolf

"Advice for those who may have leg problems. Cut off the elastic top of socks."

- Anonymous

SLEEP

"I find that the most important rule to follow is to get a minimum of 10 or more hours sleep each day. Don't let anyone discourage you from going to bed early or sleeping late in the morning, whichever works for you.

An early clue that you need to increase your sleeping time will be when your eyes fail to focus and you struggle to gain accurate location of objects. Sleep will correct the problem in a matter of hours if you just recognize what is happening.

174

Alert those around you that you have a problem and need rest. Don't ever drive a vehicle or operate even a simple piece of equipment when this occurs. Consider a clothing iron as a dangerous piece of equipment. Rest. "

Terry Fulmer from Boyertown, Pennsylvania, USA

"My wife had trouble sleeping due to restless legs and being wakened by vivid and disturbing nightmares. Fortunately this condition seems to have been fixed with a prescription from the neurologist. The Clonazepam pills have all but eliminated that problem."

- Ed and Colette from Alberta, Canada

SPEECH

"My father was having difficulty swallowing and his voice got very weak. At the time he was in rehab (after a VERY nasty fall) and the speech therapist there suggested using electro therapy (see www.vitalstim.com).

Dad was the first patient with Parkinson's to get the therapy, and it worked remarkably well. He is now getting a second set of treatments one year later. "

- Bonnie Yelverton

"One thing I was going to mention was a help for those with a weak voice. My mother was always too vain to use it that often. It is a little heavy. It straps around your waist like a fanny pack or can sit beside you in a wheelchair. It has a headset like an operator.

It's called a ChatterVox. It was wonderful when she used it. It is made by Sieman (phone 800-333-9083). I bought this about 5 years ago so they might have a better model."

- Linda McGrath from Marshfield, Massachusetts, USA

"I guess the one thing I would recommend for people with Parkinson's disease is to not forget the effects it has on your voice and swallowing. Everyone with PD needs to see a speech therapist early on in their disease. I was unaware of the effects on voice, as well as breathing (I never made the connection that simple communication kept your respiratory muscles strong).

A colleague of mine put an article in the Dallas Morning News on my desk one day regarding the Texas Voice Project. It is a group of speech therapists who are trained in the Lee Silverman Voice Treatment Program. It is subsidized by the National Parkinson's Foundation.

About 3-4 months earlier, I had stopped being able to sing a song along with the radio, which I had always done. Before long I couldn't even speak a complete sentence without being totally out of breath. My family had not told me that my voice had become so soft that they could hardly hear me. People started nodding at me, I guess to be polite, when I would ask them questions. It finally hit me after my friend put the article on my desk, that they could not hear me, and didn't want to say anything to me about it.

By the time I saw the therapist at Texas Voice Project, she told me that I should have come in about a year earlier. I was really close to being beyond help. I went through a 4 week long intensive treatment, which allowed me to regain my strength, and improve my respiratory muscle strength so that I could sing along once again with the radio.

The before and after video was amazing. They use it now as a way of fundraising for the ability to continue the project, and as a way of demonstrating the importance of speech therapy in Parkinson's patients. The goal is to have this program expand to nationwide so that all patients with PD have the ability to go through the program regardless of ability to pay.

I owe the people of Texas Voice Project my sincerest appreciation and will support their endeavor, and spread the word to make sure ALL PD patients know the importance of "thinking loud" when their perception of voice projection becomes skewed. The earlier the treatment, the better the outcome!"

Here is the contact information for Texas Voice:

Texas Voice Project for Parkinson Disease, Inc.
contact@texasvoiceproject.org
214-862-0101

- Laura Stephens, RN, CEN

SUPPORT

"I would discourage Parkinson patients from attending groups meetings, unless a very severe case is had."

- Anonymous

SWALLOWING

"I gave my mother peppermints to help her consciously swallow more frequently. I learned of the idea in some help list. However, mint can cause GRID (intestinal disorder) which can result in acid reflux. Mother was popping one right after another.

Now she uses Life Savers, butterscotch, root beer, and any candy that doesn't contain mint."

- Cori

"This is what is recommended to our clients who have issues with swallowing. We haven't needed them yet but I keep them close by. When my dad had difficulty drinking water he did these exercises and it really helped reverse his problems.

Swallowing Exercises:

- Hold tongue between teeth and swallow - 5 times
- Effortful swallow – 5 times
- Move tongue tip from front to back along the roof of your mouth – 10 times
- Stick tongue out with mouth open, do not touch lips or teeth – 10 times
- Stick out tongue without touching lips or teeth, hold for ten seconds – 5 times
- Stick out tongue and move it from corner to corner of your lips – 20 times
- Stick out your tongue and reach your chin with the tongue tip – 10 times
- Stick tongue out and up toward nose – 10 times
- Stick tongue out, pretend to lick a sucker – 10 times
- Move tongue all around lips in a circle – 10 times
- Say ka, ka, ka – 10 times
- Say ga, ga, ga – 10 times

- Push tongue to back of throat and then stick it out – 10 times
- Swallow 200 times a day
- Say "eee", high pitch, hold 15 seconds
- Push tongue in cheeks, alternating sides – 20 times
- Push tongue in cheeks, alternating sides, hold hand to resist – 10 times
- Neck stretches
- Lay flat on back, no pillow, lift head up and down – 10 times, then lift head up and hold for 10 seconds – 5 times
- Burping – 5 times
- Hold breath, hard swallow, cough – 5 times
- Pretend to gag – 5 times

- Marge Luisser

TREATMENTS/THERAPY

"Whatever my disease or condition right now, the only source of strength is my faith in God. I also believe that my suffering and trials are only meant to purify and cleanse me to be more worthy of God's unending love. I read this from a prayer to St. Therese of the Child Jesus.

I also watch comedy films and make myself as comfortable as possible. I am also gifted with a good husband who cares for me, and children and friends and relatives who continuously pray and support me. They send me letters, lots of cards and anything to comfort me.

I also tried the following therapies:

1. VAX-D therapy at the Back Pain Institute of Columbus (20 sessions)
2. Acupuncture
3. Deep Nerve Therapy Massage
4. Physical Therapy
5. Ayurvedic Medicines and oils
6. Dorn Therapy with Reiki
7. Reflexology

All these treatments helped me in dealing with my condition."

- Edna Baking

"The only suggestion I can think of that my dad would really recommend is that you have your legs massaged on a regular basis as it helps with the stiffness and helps walking with a bit more ease."

- Linda from Canada

"Recent news about research/treatment relating to Parkinson's in this part of England (Norfolk) is from the Norfolk and Norwich University hospital.

They have discovered that giving a drug via intestinal and not by mouth, direct to that part of the body, is having a dramatic effect for patients with Parkinson's.

The clip that was seen on the Eastern News TV showed two ladies who previously had been in wheel chairs walking unaided down hospital corridors.
As a consultant friend said, he thought it would be good news as the drug companies would be on to it very quickly."

- Rodney

WRITING

"When it is necessary to sign your name (or just write) make sure that your whole forearm is resting on the writing surface, not just your hand."

- David from Australia

MORE TIPS, SHORT CUTS, ADVICE
AND OBSERVATIONS

What's the one bit of advice you'd give others about Parkinson's disease?

"Keep trying!"

If you could share only one recommendation for living with Parkinson's, what would it be?

"Take your medicine regularly."

What's the greatest lesson you've learned about Parkinson's?

"There's life after Parkinson's."

Have you discovered any ways to make living with Parkinson's easier or more comfortable?

"Get and KEEP a positive attitude."

Any tips or "secrets" that helps make daily living better?

"Don't give up!"
Have you made mistakes that have set you back?

"Trying acupuncture. It didn't work."

What should we NOT do when it comes to living with Parkinson's disease?
"Listen to a non-medical doctor".

- Cale Benton Yates III

"I have had Parkinson's for 13 years. Here are my thoughts:

What's the one bit of advice you'd give others about Parkinson's disease?

"Never hide the fact that you suffer from PD. Wear this fact as a badge of honour."

If you could share only one recommendation for living with Parkinson's, what would it be?

"Do the normal things of life. Don't find an excuse not to do it because you have PD. Personally I became a student again in my sixties and studied subjects which interested me and gave me a new outlook on life. It gave me intellectual satisfaction and pride."

What's the greatest lesson you've learned about Parkinson's?

"To accept it, and lead as normal a life as you can. Value the love and affection of people close to you. They too are making sacrifices. Recognise it. I continue to go to the movies and the theatre and ballet. I don't stop doing the things I like to do because of the PD. Rather I do more of them to make life enjoyable.

I also keep a record of events and different types of activity that I undertake. I value life in a different way now. For example, I don't take it for granted and everything I get the maximum out of it. I have a desire to do a lot of things, much more than I used to have before I was ill. I also prefer to call it Parkinson's Condition rather than PD. It is not a disease as it not an infection or anything like that. It is just a different, challenging way of being."

Have you discovered any ways to make living with Parkinson's easier or more comfortable?

"We are getting a special Jensen bed which moves up and down with a motor. See www.jensenbeds.co.uk. It helps to give me a good night's sleep. I also take my medicine regularly – I don't miss it. That is quite important as one does not want to increase the dosage with all the side effects. The intellectual stimulus of my studies is a great help."

Any tips or "secrets" that helps make daily living better?

"When typing I change hands and use my left hand extensively as the PD affects the right side of my body the most. I have had shirts made for me using press studs instead of ordinary buttons which makes dressing much easier. I found a sympathetic tailor who is experimenting on this with me. I recommend him – see his website www.russellandhodge.com. This new type of press stud shirt has been copied by the tailor for a famous English actor."

Have you made mistakes that have set you back?

"I am aware when eating in a restaurant of my inability to eat neatly. I fear people staring at me. I am starting to overcome it by ignoring other people in restaurants. Normally I think to myself "I am paying good money and will eat any way I like."

Any problems or pitfalls people should watch for?

"The excess saliva secretion could be very embarrassing as it marks your clothes.

It becomes difficult to get dressed so you must allow yourself enough time to dress otherwise you could be late for something. I tend not to ask people to do things for me, even things that I would have asked people to do for me before I had PD, and this is something I must stop doing."

What should we NOT do when it comes to living with Parkinson's disease?

"Don't hide away at home and feel sorry for yourself! Don't allow yourself to become overwhelmed by the illness. Don't be excessively self-conscious when outside the home. Most people are very unobservant. Remember this. Do not allow yourself to be depressed. Life has a lot to offer even with PD."

- Ash

"Living with Parkinson's"

Walking

Concentrate on each step using a heel and toe action. Avoid doing other things at the same time such as carrying shopping bags. Shop at a supermarket where you can use a shopping trolley; you can hold on to the trolley as you are walking along.

Weight

Since you suffer that terrible feeling of tiredness, the last thing you want is to drag an overweight body around so make a special effort to slim right down such that you have no excess body weight. You will feel a lot better being a lightweight. Fitness

Stay active, go to a gym and stay for at least an hour. Do not use heavy weights. Instead, do lots of repetitions with light weights. Visit the gym at least twice a week. PD sufferers are usually older people, so take up a sport such as bowls, tennis, or golf and play at least three times a week. Do not give in to that awful feeling of tiredness. Become more active and in time you will feel the benefits. On long trips try to stop every two hours and drive in daylight as much as possible.

Sleep

You will feel much better if you sleep at least seven to eight hours per night. Sleep on your own to avoid you being disturbed and disturbing the other person by twitching and moving when you are asleep.

Alcohol seems to cause bad dreams and combined with your medication, may cause some violent reactions by you, which might harm your partner. Invest in a new mattress if your existing mattress has become distorted and uncomfortable. If you are in company tell them you need to have your sleep. Do not be afraid to be a party pooper, tell them why and they will understand.

Stress

As you know only too well, stress brings on the tremors and that awful feeling of discomfort, so make a point of avoiding stress, and do not get into protracted arguments. Stay calm when you are driving. When somebody cuts you off, it only amounts to a few extra seconds on your journey time.

If somebody pushes in front of you when you are in a queue, relax. If you have to speak in public use a chair to sit on. Use a microphone if possible, and explain why. PD suffers usually have a soft quiet voice, so in a restaurant or bar pick the quietest place so you can be easily heard and you do not have to shout as this can be very stressful.

Smoking, Alcohol, and Drugs

Your brain is no longer working properly and the last thing you should do is to reduce your brain cells, and lower its ability. Stop smoking and become teetotal; even two glasses of wine can give you that feeling the next day that you are thinking in a fog. Never ever take drugs. All of them will affect the quality of your medication.

Balance

When pulling on socks, trousers, shorts etc. lean against a wall to help with your lack of balance
Shopping

When you are accompanying someone else, walking slowly can be uncomfortable so walk quickly, or when they are in a store looking at goods and you are feeling uncomfortable standing around, find a chair and sit down until they are finished with the store.

Memory Recall

I find difficulty in using my short term memory. People's names are not retained, so use the memory key method. Say someone introduces you to a person called Bellingham, think bells and meat.

Lifestyle

Try and reduce stress in your everyday living by altering your lifestyle. Downsize your home, thus making more money available to you because of reduced costs of heating bills, electricity, rates, council tax, and maintenance.

Invest the savings to increase your income. Better still move to somewhere with a nice climate, and lower cost of living. Somewhere dry and sunny and not too humid. If you suffer from rheumatism, you will feel better in that atmosphere. There may come a time when you need help and you will be better prepared to pay the costs.

Medication

I have found that one Azilect (Rasagiline) 1 mg tablet per day combined with Sinemet or Carbilev tablets have made a distinct difference to reducing my PD symptoms.

Constipation

If it is convenient, wait for at least an hour after taking your medication to increase your control of your bowel muscles to try and defecate. Alter your diet to avoid foods that are not ideal to absorb liquid and increase your intake of fruit and vegetables.

- Reginald

"I was diagnosed in January 1999 so I'm in my eighth year and I have a few pieces of advice I would like to share.

1. Get plenty of sleep

2. Change your diet to include more fish, vegetables and fruit.

3. Arrange to see a qualified acupuncturist for a monthly session. I have been going for 8 years and it certainly makes a difference.

4. Arrange to have monthly sessions with a qualified practitioner of Reiki - it helps.

5. Visit a qualified homoeopath - I am taking medication which is helping me walk easier, and slows down "blank face" and "monotonous voice".

6. Visit a qualified chiropractor - mine keeps my spine straight and my arms and legs "balanced".

7. Swim as much as possible.

8. Don't give in to Parkinson's - you may not win the war but you will win quite a

few battles.

9. Try to avoid using a wheelchair - the more you use it the longer you will stay in it.

10. Be positive - you can make a better lifestyle for yourself.

If you met me you would not know that I suffered from Parkinson's - that's the truth."

- Brian Duffissey

"Some advice other people with Parkinson's may find helpful.

I use wheat heat packs, which are warmed in the microwave, at night to help relax tight muscles and relieve pain so that I can sleep.

I have found that water aerobics for "The Young at Heart" exercises my muscles and helps to relieve the tightness. You know the saying - "Use it or lose it!" I have found that this is true.

I take 1200mg of CoQ10 capsules daily - this has increased my energy levels. I no longer need to have a rest in the afternoons.

When I have a restless night I find that a self hypnosis CD, titled "Mind Body Healing" that I have saved to my i-pod sends me back to sleep.

Do NOT stress over small things - I have learnt that stress "hurts"- it uses up the dopamine faster.

Look after yourself. Keep positive with the knowledge that with all the research going on around the world, something will be developed soon to stop the progression of or cure Parkinson's. Keep informed of the latest research and do not lose HOPE."

- Paul Schembri from Melbourne, Australia

---

1. "I have trouble sleeping. The doctor said that the longer that I 'm up the more medications that I'll need.

2. Whenever I get upset or stressed my Parkinson's seem to get worse.

3. I have found that the more active I am the better off I am. If I sit around I get

stiff and can hardly get around.

4. When taking your standard Sinemet, make sure that you take it 1 hour before meals or 2 hours after meals. A couple of days I took my Sinemet after I ate and it took a long time for it to take effect. So please follow directions.

5. I was in the hospital for 1 and a half days in January. I took my medication with me, thankfully because the doctor didn't order any Parkinson's medication for me. I had to get really abrupt with the nurse. Finally after being late for my medications by 3 hours they let me take my own pills until the pharmacy could get them. Can you imagine what kind of condition I would have been in if I hadn't taken my pills with me?

6. I've found that my husband is in denial. He doesn't talk to me about my Parkinson's at all. He's never been to the doctor with me."

- Karen Hall

"I have noticed several things - things I have heard and read about but didn't realize how true they are:

1. Meds must come on time - on a regular basis without fail and they must come after meals to keep the person from becoming nauseated. One missed pill has a definite effect. Medicine should be given in a way to eliminate the level from dropping overnight making the morning time so much more difficult.

2. Music really makes a difference in mood and physical movement. What an important tip - one not to be ignored.
3. Keep the environment contained - one or two rooms. It is more comforting and reassuring for the family member. They do get overwhelmed with more space, more things and more feeling of responsibility.

4. MOST IMPORTANT: My father is 6'1" and I have been asking every doctor about his weight loss (including Hospice) for the last three years. I have been told it is the disease and there is nothing I could do.

I had been doing everything I could - refrigerator in the room, fruits, cereals, milk, finger type foods, everything to entice him to eat – but the Parkinson's was burning up every calorie he took in and he said food and drink did not taste good (probably because of the meds).

When he got down to 139 lbs and I went ballistic the doctor finally took me seriously and put Dad on an appetite enhancing drink called Megace. He got 1 drink in the morning and 1 at night. I had to discontinue the one at night because he was literally up all night eating. He has gained 16 lbs in two months and for whatever reason is enjoying his food. He is gaining strength, his bowels are so much better because he is getting volume. It is the single best thing I have done. I believe it is a must but I am only a daughter, not a doctor. They have to have some weight to have strength and stamina and food in their stomach to go with all those pills. We also use anti-nausea pills on a daily basis and that has stopped the nausea that the medicine causes."

- Melody from Texas, USA

"My older brother John, who was diagnosed with PD about 6 years before I was, has always been my mentor, my idol, my hero. I could go on and on. When I finally was diagnosed in 2001 he was the first person I called for advice.

After answering many questions for me I asked him if there was only one piece of advice he could offer what it would be. He said: *"Learn to cope and don't dwell on it."* His words echo in my head each time I experience a new or different symptom for the first time, and each time I get frustrated with my buttons or mad at my knife and fork. Every time I repeat them to myself, they seem to make more sense."

- Anonymous

"Firstly, I'm Bryn Davies, 51 years old from Truro in Cornwall, UK. I have had PD since I was 36 years old. An ex Military Warrant Officer I am now no longer fit to take a paid job. I will be delighted to give you a few tips:
The first one is on medication instructions. If people read them it could scare them half to death. People must know that of the many, many side effects listed they may get one or 2 but generally speaking most will get no side effects from many of the drugs.

The second is, when you freeze you tend to fall on your knees so buy a set of knee protectors like the kids wear for skate boarding. They don't cost much and will save you ruining your knees.

Number three. If you have a weak bladder and go to the loo through the night, instead of putting the light on and waking your partner up, buy some of the luminous stars (the ones you put on children's ceilings) and put them on the floor for you to follow in the dark.

Read as much as you can about PD and the medication that is prescribed because you will know what is happening and what medication the doctor can prescribe to help.

If possible try to be seen by a PD specialist because a GP is just that; a 'General' Practitioner, not a PD specialist.

 If you see someone with PD having a bad time of it, don't panic. It may never happen to you as everyone with PD is so different.

If you have young children in the house or just visiting, don't take your medication out of the packaging until you need it.

If you cannot open the child proof bottles that your medication comes in, just give it to a child, the child will do it for you.

That's it for now, but tell everyone that with all the research going that one day we will all say;

I USED TO HAVE PARKINSON'S DISEASE."

- Bryn Davis from Truro, Cornwall, United Kingdom

"I have had PD since I was 47 or about 5 years. I don't take Sinemet but take Selegilene and that's all. I have turned to holistic medicine and a healthier lifestyle because of PD.

I see a NUCCA chiropractor (National Upper Cervical Care Association) that for me has made a big difference. I've seen regular chiropractors and had some relief but this specialist has made a big difference.

At first I read everything and subscribed to many different info sites. I found that after awhile I was very discouraged reading about what may happen to me and decided I would research various ways to help myself.

I have a wonderful neurologist that listens to me and doesn't just start prescribing medicines. If your doctor won't listen to you and your symptoms, find someone who will!

Everyone has different concerns with PD and taking a new drug for each new problem is NOT the answer. Realize that you may have to live with some problems and adapt.

I ask lots of questions and talk to lots of PD patients to see what works for them. It appeared to me that those who were most active involved in making their own decisions and keeping a positive attitude were the ones progressing slowly and doing the best. So I started looking into what I had to do to make my body the best it could be.

I explored diets and after realizing I was generally doing worse if I ate a lot of meat, I looked into vegetarian diets. I found The Hallelujah diet online and because I believe God truly maps everything for us in His Word, the Bible, I decided to apply its principles to my body and intake and what a difference it makes for me.

I am not a religious practiser (as I munch on a Valentine Chocolate) but just the few changes in diet I have made have helped tremendously. I have done a cleansing diet (made more difference) and have turned my home into a green clean and have been eliminating as many chemicals as I can.

I refuse any medication that isn't natural except Selegiline because it may be a neuro protective agent. I don't take supplements. Waste of money! I take natural remedies for colds and problems and they may work a bit slower but I feel so much healthier and they work.

I understand how my body works and how what I put into it and do to it affects it. Sure I'm concerned that I won't last 10 more years at my Assistant Teaching position until I can retire at 62 but I do the best I can, even teaching myself to write left handed.

Mostly I stay active, positive and rested and when I have the opportunity to help those newly diagnosed or having problems I encourage them to not give in. Our bodies change as we get older and most naturally adapt or find new ways of doing old things to cope. Just because I am not 'old' why should I give in to PD? The body renews itself every 3 months and I can make my body better, maybe not perfect, even if it's in small ways.

The greatest lesson I have learned from PD? Medical doctors don't know everything and putting a drug into your body has consequences, mostly bad. Buy stock in drug companies, they con everybody and may make you rich, at the expense of the world's health. The body can and wants to heal itself.

Best advice? Get silky PJ's to help you move in bed. Get lots of rest. De-stress your life as much as you can.

Best recommendation? Learn all you can about you and your body. Don't be afraid to see a holistic specialist. See a NUCCA chiropractor and nutritionist. Do things that make you happy. Stay active. Make your husband vacuum and above all believe in prayer and do it!

What you should not do is give into PD. You are not PD you are still you. Don't be ashamed if you shake or slur words or are incontinent. Yes, it's unfortunate but you are not dead.

My husband constantly tells people that I'm the best back scratcher there is when I shake and it makes me and others laugh. So I don't hand write letters and cards anymore, big deal! I now TELL people how I feel and I use a check card instead of writing checks and I'm the worst badminton player but I was never great.

In closing, focus on you, not PD or what it is or may do to you, but how you can make you the best you can be."

- Gail from Long Lake, New York, USA

"Shortcuts for Parkies"

"I'm in Stage 2-3 of the "postural" type of Parkinson's as opposed to the type that starts out with a tremor. I live alone and have had to develop some new habits which I'd like to share with you. If your symptoms differ from mine, perhaps you can adapt some of these to your own needs. Here are the measures I've taken that have been most valuable to me:

1. Keeping a daybook. If you have any trouble remembering things - important conversations, appointments, etc., I recommend this practice. Buy a notebook in the size of your choice, lined or unlined. Mine is full size (roughly 8.5 x 11), college ruled. Plan to devote a full page to each day. Write the date at the top, then jot down that day's "to-do" list. As you progress through your list of tasks, make any notes you want to remember.

For example:

- Wash purple socks separately in cold water!!! (uh-oh!)
- Neurologist appt. switched to (date)
- I owe Dorothy $10.00

You can also use your day page for keeping track of any aspects of your medication such as dosage schedule, side effects, effectiveness, etc.

Jot down a recipe, website, etc. that you hear on the radio.
Try writing a haiku.
Balance your bank account.

Practice your handwriting. And by the way, if writing by hand is no longer an option, and if you can type, the daybook will easily translate to computer use.

There is nothing sacred about a daybook except the need to use it daily! If you do, you'll probably find yourself referring back to it often for info that might otherwise have slipped your mind. When you fill up a daybook, be sure to have a new one ready. Write the inclusive dates of the full one on the front (many covers will not retain ink, so you may need to use matte-finish tape) and save it for possible future reference. You may never refer to it, but as the saying goes, "If you

190

throw it away, you'll need it next day."

It will be very helpful to keep your daybook with you wherever you go. Having found this harder to remember at home than when I go out, I would often end up answering the phone in the bedroom, reaching for my book, and recalling I'd left it in the kitchen. This led me to form another habit:

2. Keeping a carrier. Especially for those of us who have difficulty walking, a carrier is a godsend. I have attached an inexpensive wire tray to my walker; it happens to fit perfectly between the handles. On it, at all times, I keep my daybook, a pen, reading glasses, and my cell phone.

Your carrier may be a canvas tote bag, or a basket attached to your scooter. However, a tray has the added advantage of standing at the ready when you need to clear a coffee cup, snack plate, etc. from the deck, the desk, or anywhere else you like to nosh. I'm an inveterate computer snacker, and without a carrier next to my desk it would soon look more like an untidy kitchen counter.

3. Here's a tip for pet owners, especially new kittens or puppies: I'm breaking in two mischievous kittens. In training them to stay off the counters and my desk, I found the tried-and-true methods (shaking a can of pennies, spritzing with water) not at all convenient, since my chosen deterrent was never at hand when I needed it.

I now wear a very loud coach's whistle on a cord around my neck. Cats hate loud noises, and they absolutely despise this whistle. I'm not fond of the sound either, but I soon hope to have them reacting even when I reach for the whistle so I won't have to actually use it.

4. Proactive problem solving. Having had a little success with self-styled solutions, I'm now encouraged to face logistical problems head on instead of simply enduring the way things are. Of course I sometimes get stuck, as I am with the problem of 20-lb boxes of cat litter--hard to lift and awkward to handle. But I'm working on it."

- Maggie Mangan from St. Louis, Missouri, USA

"Well I think that the most positive things to do concerning my PD are exercising, reading (which I do a lot), and if you can, try to get out as much as possible. As I only have started PD I really don't have much to say about it, except that I try to think positive things, and try to smile and laugh as much as I can.

I hope this helps someone, as I know I will get worse as time goes on."

- Mildred

"I tend to try and forget that I've got Parkinson's and take each day as it comes and try to have something to look forward to. Also to laugh when I can't get up from the chair!

Speaking of getting up I gear myself up to have a big surge of energy and then jump up – this works most of the time!! Getting up from a settee is different. I rock backward and forward to gain momentum.

When I have trouble swallowing tablets I take a mouthful of water and then take a deep breath to relax the throat and then swallow."

- Gillian

"One thing that I have learned is that with PD I get a lot of anxiety, and as a hunter fisherman, trail hiker, it bothers me. I think I am lost, so I have a GPS that I carry. They are less expensive now days. A good thing to have."

- Anonymous

"A week ago I traveled to Colorado to attend 4 days of meetings of a service organization on whose Board I serve. The days were long, and the meetings intense. I was pleased that physically I was able to participate well, and the PD limitations didn't seem more than an annoyance of the tremor and awareness of reduced energy level.

Then I arrived back home and crashed. Now 14 days later I'm still recovering, and haven't gotten the balance back to what it was before.

I didn't understand what had happened to make these past 14 days so miserable, until I was reading a book "Parkinson's Disease" (Reducing Symptoms with nutrition and drugs) by Drs. Geoffrey & Lucille Leader.

I had read in many articles that stress was a problem. Now I know why.

'Dopamine also influences the control of stress-related symptoms. Stress requires the body to produce adrenaline and the adrenal glands manufacture this hormone--FROM DOPAMINE!' And we know that deficiency of dopamine is Parkinson's disease.

So by drawing 4 days of adrenaline for my meetings, when I came off the adrenaline "high", the result was not fun! I did not know that adrenaline is manufactured in our brains from dopamine. My meetings obviously depleted the limited supply my brain is producing now, and used all the medication I am

192

taking as well.

Bottom line - if I allow or encounter situations that call for adrenaline, I know that I will suffer serious consequences.

And that was a good lesson to learn."

- Carl

"A few tips:

1. Keep stress level low.
2. Keep mind active.
3. Keep body active.
4. Lead an active life where possible.
5. Don't talk when eating.
6. Use smooth peanut butter if you choke.
7. Don't over protect the person and allow them space."

- Jenny

"We have learned as we go along certain things which had been very helpful.

1. We bought a recliner chair that goes all the way up into a standing position. This is very helpful because after a nap the bradykinesia makes it very difficult to stand and become mobile

2. We ordered some foam handled cutlery from Rolyan (1-630-226-0000) which makes eating so much easier.

3. We have a bedside commode, as it becomes difficult to make it to the bathroom as the muscles just don't get going quick enough. Also, pull-ups are helpful to avoid accidents.

4. We need to constantly remind him to use the bathroom on a long trip and to move and stay loose.

5. Being closed in the house for long periods of time causes severe boredom and depression and getting out even for a short ride in the car, or pulling up to a drive-in Dunkin doughnuts is a terrific mood elevator. Actually caffeine is very beneficial to these patients!
6. We installed a shower in the house that one can roll into without having to climb in the tub.

7. Using a walker and a cane is very helpful for stability.

8. A wheelchair is occasionally necessary.

9. Driving is out of the question once mobility is an issue. This can cause severe depression especially in men. It represents a loss of independence like nothing else. However if the muscles are not responding quickly, something jumping into the road such as a child, could be a disaster. Explaining it in that way to him made all the difference.

10. Using the word Parkinson's I find is not helpful. The stigma attached to this disease makes it very scary. We tried to downplay the clinical terms and deal with the symptoms that we can treat. Unfortunately my father knows several people who have Parkinson's who have been alive for many years and have lived to the end stages. Their wives also took such good care of them that they lived it out to the bitter end. This is scary for my father to think of.

11. Having different people come to the house even for one to two hours is incredibly helpful. The afflicted tends to become resentful of their caretakers especially if they are family members. It is amazing how much more energy and motivation we see in my father when someone new shows up.

12. We get depressed when he just sits in his chair with that vacant look. We have 5 children in our family. It is very helpful for us to maintain our own network of support. We email each other regularly for updates. We have also suffered with our own depression watching this process take place. However, despite it all, my father will tell you at every day is a gift.

When he was in rehab, they had a party for Mardi Gras and all the patients in the long-term care facility attended. When he looked around and saw what other people looked like, he began to realize that he was still very fortunate.

13. My parents are very religious but are not able to get out for church, so it has been helpful to have a visit from a Catholic nun to the house for communion."

- Kristen Kratzert

"My tips are:

1. Kitchen tools to help chop and slice fruit and vegetables. There are various gadgets that can be found in kitchen shops; Lakeland Plastics in UK; Tchibo mail order catalogue.

2. Shoes, sandals and winter boots with Velcro / touch closing fastenings rather than laces.

3."Touch" bedside light so you don't have to fiddle with switches in the dark.

4. For my bicycle I am going to buy adult stabilizers and a dual brake lever so I can operate both front and back brakes from one lever on my "good" side. The stabilizers are quite expensive but I'm sure will be justified by the increased mobility especially when on holiday. These items are from www.bikecare.co.uk and www.disabledcycling.2s.com.

5. In crowded places I try to leave some space in front of me and concentrate while taking deep breaths. I'm not worried now about asking for help and everyone has been very understanding."

- Carol from Cornwall, United Kingdom

"I have difficulty opening plastic bags that are sealed after opening such things as cheeses. My solution was to get 2 small rubber grippers and grab each side with these. Actually, this is the ONLY way I can open them.

I learned to carry straws in my purse after being caught a few times where no straw was available, such as visiting in someone's home. Too many days I cannot drink from a cup or a glass.

Spacing my activity each and every day is a must. If I have to go for an appointment or shop a bit, I plan to take a brief rest immediately upon returning home.

I have such a fluctuation in temperature tolerance. I use lightweight (but warm) bedding and keep several items arranged so that I can easily pull the layers that I need at any time without having to get up.

With so many people NOT understanding PD and what a person lives with, I have pretty much given up on trying to explain/educate past a certain point.

Staying away from stress is crucial! Although it may seem anti-social, I have to excuse myself from situations not only with my family, but also with friends. Stress is definitely a factor in exacerbating symptoms and sometimes is responsible for actually putting me in bed!"

- Anonymous

ENCOURAGEMENT AND INSPIRATION

"There is nothing funny about Parkinson's but funny things happen to people with Parkinson's.

For instance, did hear what the Parkinson's passenger said to the flight attendant?.....What turbulence? Or since getting a treadmill because of Parkinson's I'm losing weight and eating better. Not because of the treadmill but because only half the food gets to my mouth!

My girlfriend says I'm going through the joke stage of Parkinson's and I do like to tell this joke whenever I feel the need to tell someone I have Parkinson's. Having Parkinson's is not so bad in fact I had a chance to meet Michael J. Fox........ Ya, but our hands would not meet! I didn't really meet Mr. Fox but the joke puts others at ease about my shaky hand. And the more nervous I am the more my hand shakes so the jokes help me be less nervous especially in social settings."

- Dan Thomas from San Diego, USA, Parkinson's since '04

"I don't know if I'm the best person to be giving anyone advice about how to deal with Parkinson's in view of the fact that I am relatively new to the disease myself, I was diagnosed four years ago at age 56.

What's the one piece of advice I would give to anyone who is new to the condition? That's easy. I would say to them, "Avoid like the plague the misery guts of this world."

You know the type. He's easy enough to spot. He's got negativity oozing from every pore of his dreary personality. I'm sure it's the same in the US as it is here in the UK but you walk in the door of your friendly local pub and there he is.

He is usually either standing at the bar boring the hind legs off some poor unfortunate soul with his morbid tales of death and ill health or he is seated by himself being avoided by the more alert who don't want to be drawn into his doleful web of misery. His glass is always half empty, never half full.

If you should feel sorry for him and make the mistake of asking him how he is you'll always get the same reply, 'Aah not too bad.' And this when you can see that he is clearly as fit as a fiddle and as well fed as a butchers dog. After a few minutes in his clutches all you want to do is run outside and throw yourself under the nearest truck, just to get some relief.

That's enough about Old Misery Guts. I prefer to spend my time in the company of more positively minded humorous people.

A few more thoughts before I put the PC away for another day.

Sometimes, more often in the afternoon, I have a bit of trouble swallowing. The remedy, chew a piece of gum or suck on a boiled sweet. Works for me!!

Enjoy a pint of beer, or two!! Not on your own, in good company.

Take up golf. I started playing golf twenty five years ago. It's a great game and you meet nice people. I was never that good at it but it's fun trying.

Get out in the fresh air for a brisk walk. What harm can it do!

Mistakes I've made, one springs to mind. I was getting ready to go out to a formal dinner with some friends who were due to pick me up at four o'clock. As the hour approached and I attempted to insert my cufflinks into the double cuffs of my shirt my hands began to tremble and the more I fumbled the more I trembled. In the end I had no alternative but to await the arrival of my friends and seek assistance, much to their amusement. They made me buy large brandy's all around.

Lesson.....Make a mental note of the fumbly bits and allow yourself more time. It's cheaper in the long run!!"

- Michael Kerr from Redbourn, Herts, United Kingdom

"Two years ago I decided to join my local gym to see if it could help. And I have to say it is the best thing I've done in my eight years with P.D. I attend five days a week. I do forty minutes cardio vascular exercise i.e. 20 minutes each on the treadmill and 20 minutes on the bike. I then work out on two or three resistance machines. I do another session of c/v exercise. At the beginning and end of the session I warm up/ cool down with stretch exercises. Presently, I am unable to exercise because I have had a pacemaker fitted and I cannot wait to get back

The other benefit of going to the gym is the social interaction with other gym members and the instructors. I have gained a lot of respect from them because I refuse to give in to my situation. Added to this I find if you think positive and get on with life people are very supportive but if you are miserable and full of self pity they just back off.

A further insight I have learned is to live for the day and the moment rather than looking back to the past or worrying about the future. I also have discovered that it is best to live within my limitations. It is best step back and take things easy if I'm having a bad day. Otherwise I only find myself frustrated and don't gain

197

anything by it.

Whenever I meet someone I have not met before I tell them straight away that I have P.D. This avoids them making wrong judgments and by and large I find people are very understanding. And very often they will tell me someone in their family has had the disease. This makes them even more understanding. I have also found the majority of people are very kind and helpful. Very often they will offer help even before I ask for it.

Finally, I gain great strength from my Christian faith. I have a degree in theology but I learned more about myself and my God in the time I have had PD than I ever did in my three years studying theology. I believe we grow best in our suffering rather than when life is a bed of roses."

- George Cawood

"Having had Parkinson's for over 10 years now I offer the following thoughts and suggestions.

1. Take as much control of your life with Parkinson's as you can. The mind is an incredibly powerful tool and most of us can control our thoughts and attitudes much more than we realize.

Shakespeare wrote "There is nothing either good or bad, but thinking makes it so". In other words we can choose how we are going to respond to having Parkinson's. For example, by deciding to focus on what we can do, and feeling good about that, rather than let the negatives get us down. Positive thinking really can affect the way we feel both emotionally and physically.

2. Learn to laugh at yourself and encourage your partner to laugh with you. Humor is used a lot in war time to belittle the enemy. Parkinson's is one of our enemies and if, for example, we can laugh at ourselves when we walk in an unusual way (as if we were doing it on purpose) then the enemy can be cut down to size.

3. Be your own Parkinson's expert. Read as much about it as you can. Look up the research (including the meaning of the obscure words!). Many GP's are not able to keep up the latest research and developments in Parkinson's. They don't have the time - but often we do.

It helps us feel less of a victim and more in charge of our destiny. Every new trick we learn ups our spirits and puts us in charge. Knowing more of what new medications and approaches are available puts us in partnership with our medical practitioners. No doctor worth his salt will think we are trying to be clever. They will applaud our efforts to manage our disease in the most effective way.

4. When walking gets difficult I find my small electronic portable metronome very useful - its loud click usually gets me started and of course I can vary the speed!"

- John Goodwin

"Here's an easy thing to do: Never, never ever lose your sense of humor. If you don't have a sense of humor go get one

Remember, "Where there's no sense there's no feeling."

Laughs are ever so much cheaper than all these dopey drugs."

- Jerry

"My one tip is to hang in there and never give up hope.

My brother Billy who has Parkinson's disease was really, really ill as his medication had gone awry. He was hospitalized for two months after being cared for at home 24/7 for one month. He was really ill, totally out of it, and couldn't walk, dress, wash, or eat without assistance.

Thanks to the persistence of the medical team and lots of loving encouragement from the family, Billy is living at home and more independent than ever. His dopamine intake is doubled; I put on the Neupro every 24 hours.

Billy lives a very independent life now; I just keep a watchful eye. He now walks unaided about 2 to 3 miles daily.

His mood has lifted and his outlook is positive. My advice is get the medication monitored preferably under medical supervision. As a caregiver I had to stand back sometimes reluctantly as I was anxious if Billy wanted to go walking without me. But gradually I let go and he's going further.

Billy was discharged from hospital on the 7th July 2006 and we've had the best quality 8 months that I can remember. Every day is a new day and where there's life there's hope. I thought this time last year I would be in mourning in 2007, but instead Billy and I are celebrating life together. Of course Billy hates the Parkinson's but he loves life more."

- Anonymous

"Don't give up. Do what you can as long as you can. On top of 10 year old Parkinson's, I had a stroke. Now, at age 91, unable to stand or take a step, I get around in an electric wheel chair in a life-care community and still do as much for myself as I can. Focus on what you have left not on what you have lost. Consciously sweep negative thoughts out of your mind and be thankful."

- Verna S. Winstead

"I guess if I were going to say anything about Parkinson's, it would be this: for anyone who has this disease, I believe strength is the most important component that we have and we must put it into practice constantly and never give in to weakness.

Strength of body, strength of mind and soul is vitally important. These things are important for anyone in any situation, but especially for those of us who find ourselves fighting this weakening disease.

I could give in to this tomorrow and just stop trying to live a normal life, and I would probably be dead in a very short time. But I choose to fight it and do everything in my power to stay one step ahead of it. I stay as busy as possible, as involved as possible. I don't know that this will help, but that is where I am right now."

- Anonymous

"My name is Robert. I'm 53 years old and currently residing in Durham, NC. I was diagnosed with PD in 1998. I was on three different meds; Requip, Sinemet and Amantadine. I say was because after attending a healing service at my church I have now been totally and completely off all meds for approximately 4years. My doctors at Duke continue to be rather perplexed about my situation. I continue to have rather mild symptoms but no progression. I have been on occasion sharing my testimony with GlaxoSmithKline drug reps who supply doctors with medications for the treatment of PD.

Jesus is still the great physician."

- Robert

"All I can say about my wife Barbara who was diagnosed with Parkinson's 7 years ago when she was 50, is that in many ways the news inspired her to try things that she (probably) wouldn't otherwise have done.

She attended Art college when she was young so already had a background in painting. She decided to try to work using glass and has had some success, in that her work has been exhibited at a Harrogate Art festival during the last two summers. Also, a new gallery opened in Newcastle and she has exhibited there.

She has sold a number of her creations and met a whole new group of people. She was asked if she would allow some of her work to be auctioned for charity; this she has done (successfully) twice. We are now looking for a kiln to progress her work, as a new gallery in North Shields is opening soon and she has been asked to exhibit there, as well as being given shared use of a studio. She has rediscovered her love of painting as well and has produced a number of canvases.

Obviously Barbara has her share of bad days - indeed she recently had an operation to help with her walking - but I feel that her story is inspiring.

Hopefully, when I retire in May I can take a more active role in what she does."

- Richard

"I do have a few items of advice to share. First and foremost, never, ever forget your primary caregiver or take them for granted. Too often, it is the Parkinson's patient who is "made over". Your caregiver is there for you and your caregiver is going through just about the same situation as you. Remember your caregiver and give thanks everyday for what they do.

Next, do not be ashamed or embarrassed by your Parkinson's. Let those around you know what you are going through and how you feel. Open up to your co workers and let them be apart of your treatment. It is up to us Parkinson's patients to educate the public on the disease."

- Greg Gardner from Yuma, Arizona, USA

"My husband is taking only one prescription. I try alternative ways of dealing with his Parkinson's. I am always looking for something that may help. I know there's a cure for it, but finding it is the question.

I give him a good vitamin/mineral supplement. He eats well, sleeps good, and most of the time, he is in good spirits. First of all, I don't deny that he's ill, but we laugh anyway. He's naturally jolly, and has a zest for life, even in his condition.

I lay hands on him throughout the day, quote scriptures and believe for a healing. I give him lots of vitamin C (1000mg) capsules from Swanson's vitamins as they're very reasonably priced. Vitamin B6 is good.

He has a great mind, great memory, very focused. We act like he doesn't have anything wrong with him. We still talk and act like everything is okay, and for us, it has to be that way, because we know that God will never leave us or forsake us.

'Yea, though I walk through the valley of the shadow of death, I will fear no evil, for thou art with me, thy rod and thy staff, they comfort me. Surely goodness and mercy shall follow me all the days of my life, and I will dwell in the house of the lord forever.'

Read psalms 91 over and over and believe what it says. And if you don't know Christ as your personal savior, receive him today and believe his word.

I'm believing for a miracle.

My husband will be 75 in August, and considering all things, he's doing well.

I don't give him much dark meat. He eats mostly white meats, fish, chicken, turkey, tuna, salmon, and mackerel. Lots of fruits and vegetables. He has a great appetite.

I'm thinking about taking him to the chiropractor when the weather fairs up. Getting his spine back in balance, and I even believe physical therapy would help, if you're up to it. I just wish I had started earlier on.

Quote scripture, and never loose hope. Remember psalms 91 as much as you can. 'Faith cometh by hearing, and hearing by the word of God.'

He said all things are possible if we only believe."

- Faye from West Virginia, USA

"I think the most helpful thing is being open and honest with others in your life about your condition. I feel prayer is vital to help keep yourself grounded in what is really important in the long "eternal" things in life.

Exercise has helped me keep mobile and strong mentally and helped me to physically keep moving. Don't put yourself in a box of thinking if something happens to one person with Parkinson's that's what will happen to you. As a medical provider no two people ever have exactly the same reaction to any disease.

Keep your faith, family and friends close and know God will heal you one day either here or in heaven. Bless all of you."

- Victoria

"My philosophy is: live each day at a time - if you can only do small things, do them well. Don't give up doing something because you *think* you can't do it anymore; be happy if you *can* still do it!"

- Joanne

"The one hint that I can give anyone that has Parkinson's is to get up and live life, go to work and make the best of your situation. Give yourself to someone that needs more help than you do. Laugh at yourself and your clumsy ways and if you are lucky enough to have a grandchild who needs more help than you, give your help.

Enjoy your life. Get your children around you and be happy with your lot in life. No one deserves to be sick but Parkinson's is not cancer and we can live with it and still have a meaningful existence.

I tell my children to take me to the nursing home when I am ready and I will love it. I can make the best of any situation. Don't get overwhelmed with your situation. Remember, it could be worse. Look on the bright side; you're still here and breathing. Laugh, Laugh, Laugh.

If you are a sad sack no one will want to be with you. My children who are 40, 34, and 25 come home a lot to have a home cooked meal and to have a day of laughter, since we have been a laughing family forever. They also come to see their mom, and I am grateful for them and so grateful that they want to see me.

Stop feeling sorry for yourself and move on to something happier. Watch a good comedy, read a funny book or read a tearjerker that will also make you realize that your life is not so bad.

I love to play FreeCell on the computer. I love my computer and I love TV and all the new shows. I have TiVo so I am always taping shows to watch in my spare time. I love to read and have a book swap at the beauty parlor so other people can enjoy what I read. I belong to all kinds of book clubs and love to own books (am running out of space). I love the crossword puzzle in my local paper and the jumble keeps my brain going. I love to talk to people (typical hairdresser).

I love life....I don't love Parkinson's but we all have to get something and I feel that it is the lesser of evils."

- Sue Drummond

"The things that have helped me the most would be my faith in the Lord, the love and support of my husband and the positive attitude that I try to obtain on a daily basis doing the things that I still can do and not focusing on my limitations.

We still have our Parkie moments, (tears and laughter), but concentrating on the positive and loving the Lord can be our saving grace. Keeping family close and in our prayers is another positive step in my daily walk with Parkinson's."

- Jan and Andy Strachan from Leduc, Alberta, Canada

"About the best advice I can offer to people who are experiencing symptoms of Parkinson's disease is NOT to settle with them or "learn how to be comfortable with them". That is not possible!

I was diagnosed with PD in 1998. I am now into the most active time of research concerning overcoming it than I have ever been. I would recommend reading a book called "Hope Heals: How One Man Conquered Parkinson's" by William P. Hansen, and "What Your Doctor May Not Tell You About Parkinson's Disease" by Jill Marjama-Lyons, M.D., an electronic book "Parkinson's Disease: The Greatest American Blunder" by Noel N. Batten, also "Radical Forgiveness" by Colin Tipping, and "A Course In Miracles". Also books by Caroline Myss, Ph.D. There are numerous others.

I recommend that people start believing in miracles. I recommend that they listen to their doctors with a grain of salt, and at the same time seek help from alternative sources, such as acupuncture, Charkra balancing, vitamins and supplements, particular essential sugars and Glutathione.

There are many resources out there, they tend to be expensive and it takes time and research to discern what works best for you. It is a difficult journey. I feel strongly though, that there is a reason for it and that the outcome need not be to simply learn to live with it, but to grow with it and hopefully overcome it."

- Diane Lamas

"It gets very discouraging at times, but you have to have a sense of humor. One day I was going to the basement to check on my kitty. Like most people who have this illness, sometimes you can't slow down and the next thing I knew I was laying on the floor with my face in the cat's food bowl and water dish. Trust me; it was a sight to see.

There have been other times when I can find no humor whatsoever. I've fallen on my right shoulder so often that now I have a torn rotator cuff.

I use a walker most of the time. I have a cane and a scooter also. I think the one that has helped me the most is the walker."

- Kathryn Kinsella

"Simplify by getting rid of as much stuff as you can. Not easy but very worthwhile. I'm still working on this. Clutter just slows everyone down more and leads to irritability and accidents.

Try to encourage your loved one with PD to explain what they are going through. Otherwise, you might feel impatient due to a lack of understanding. Some people don't say much and that makes cooperating with them more difficult.

Keep walking if at all possible."

- Eileen from California, USA

"I find if I keep myself occupied I don't feel so bad because I am concentrating on the task instead of thinking that I don't feel well."

- Elizabeth from England

"The best advice I got was from my neurologist who told me to look at Parkinson's as only one part of my life, not all of my life and not who I am."

- Anonymous

"My # 1 top advice: as a newly diagnosed recipient of Parkinson's I felt like I was the only one alarmed by the news. My primary care M.D. detected it first and seemed very calm about it. He referred me to a neurologist.

She didn't act like I should be overly concerned either. At that time I didn't know anything about it or if a person could die from it. That is when I started my own research and found "All About Parkinson's" on the internet along with other sources of information.

My advice would be to get educated and keep up-dated on everything you can learn about the disease."

- Anonymous

"The person affected with PD may seem to be pushing him/herself too hard. It is a common reaction and it is all right to push yourself. The more active you are the longer it will take for your body to slow down. Your body is the only one that will tell you when to call it a day's work!"

- Dee from Gatineau, Quebec, Canada

"I find that keeping a positive outlook on life helps. Do all the things you wish to do, don't let your shaky hands stop you from going to a restaurant for instance. So what if your peas fall from your fork. Laugh at it and all your friends will laugh with you and that in itself will make you feel more comfortable.

Don't even listen to or read about tales of woe about other peoples PD that can be depressing. Just find your own way of living with it, and keep taking the tablets!!"

- Dave M.

"I think it is very important to look for the positive and smile and really laugh a lot. It is commonly believed in the medical field that good belly laughs are good for your health. I have friends who every day email me funny stories, etc. and I look for funny shows on TV."

- Wilma Schmerer from Walla Walla

"When my Father was first diagnosed with Parkinson's my family thought we were going to lose him. We constantly babied him and did everything for him. This only made him worse.

Then we got him in home therapy and starting playing games with him such as checkers, cards etc. He really enjoyed this .We also starting getting him out more and making him do stuff for himself. He showed a big improvement.

They got his Parkinson medicine regulated and today you would not even know that he had Parkinson's. He shuffles still a little bit and his right arm shakes a little at all times but this is a miracle compared to where he was a long time ago. At first he could not walk or feed himself. He was confined to a wheel chair or bed.

I thank God everyday for his wonderful healing powers. I also want to thank the great doctors for their knowledge and continual research on Parkinson."

- Jeannette Shilling from Roanoke, Virginia, USA

"We have a very close friend who was diagnosed last year at the age of 60. The disease is progressing faster than we had hoped, but he is taking it in his stride.

One of the things he thrives on is being with people who share his love of humor and laughter, so a group of us get together several times a week to share our hilarious experiences gained from just living.

After all, one must have a sense of humor just to get through this life. He and a friend who also has Parkinson's look forward greatly to these times and we all feel we are helping somehow."

- Anonymous

"Living with Mr. Parkinson for the past 12 to 14 years, I hope that the following has some merit:

Billiards is my hobby. Now my hobby and Parkinson's don't mix but the other day in a game of 9 ball I made the 5 ball run out. There was that ray of sunshine - enjoy it.

Parkinson's affects (I believe) concentration - fight it. The disease takes a toll the body configuration - don't let Pride keep you at home.

Keep informed which will help you and your doctor communicate."

- Charles D Mills, AKA Dury

"Stay away from Diet Coke - I felt much better after I did!

Surround yourself with positive people and try as much as possible to keep a cheerful, positive attitude. The term "fake it till you make it" applies here.

Find a neurologist that you "click" with and who really listens to you - this helps you get the best possible care and your medicine in the right dosage.

LAUGH!! Laughter is the best medicine.

A glass of red or white wine in the evening seems to really help also."

- Anonymous

"If I were to give only one bit of advice to anyone who has been diagnosed with Parkinson's, it would be simply to have, and keep, a good attitude about life and all that is happening to you. I believe that one's attitude determines so much in life.

I recently read this:

"Ability determines what you are able to do in life.
 Motivation determines what you will do in life.
 Attitude determines how well you do it."

If I am allowed to give a little more advice, I would say that we need to remember that no two cases of Parkinson's are exactly alike. No matter who you see or know with PD, or what you hear or read about PD, you are not necessarily going to be like that or have happen to you what has happened to them, because you are unique and so is each case of PD.

And, going a little further, I would also like to say to anyone with PD to always remember that a cure can come at any time, so just be hopeful that it does come soon; take each day as it comes; think positively; and pray a lot."

- Nancy Fox

"What could I tell someone else about this disease is to be patient. We take it one day at a time, and deal with whatever develops as it develops. We have our good days and we have days that are not so good.

Dizziness or what my husband calls dizziness is something we're dealing with right now. Talking is also something we do a lot of and I think that this is a very good thing. Sharing fears and concerns and working together to find answers or solutions if you will to these problems is good therapy for both of us."

- Anonymous

----

1. When your legs start to cramp or ache, go into the shower and turn on the water to as hot as you can stand it. This helps to stop those nasty cramps and aches that keep you up all night.

 2. When I am unable to sleep because of the Parkinson's, I get up out of my bed and either read, go on the computer or listen to a CD on my CD player with earphones that delivers a soft and whispering sounds from the "Ocean Waves" or a lovely "Brook' that is traveling down a stream. I also do picture places of total beauty, while doing so. Milk is another sleep helper because it contains a sleep ingredient and this is what helps babies sleep.

 3. I keep away from ALL stressful situations, such as, TV programs, families that argue etc. I try to keep myself calm at all given times. I have found that when my stress level goes up, so does my shaking and leg weakness as well as my balance.

 4. Keeping active is so very, very important for my "depression" and the movement disorder or I start to stiffen up bad. Water therapy has been a great help to me. I also bought a "three wheel tricycle" to ride so that I am able to balance myself when riding. I ride slow and visit my neighbors and enjoy the Florida sun on nice days.

5. My attitude has to be one of "don't let it beat you, you beat it" This is so important from what I have seen in the Parkinson's meetings. I have seen others that have just given up and live each day in a riding scooter, wheel chair and do nothing from day to day. They are the ones that this movement disorder will bring them down fast.

It is not a killer disease, nor is it a disease that will totally cripple you, IF you work to keep it at bay and do all you can to slow the process down. I am now seventy three and have had Parkinson's for some time, yet, here I sit with steady hands and fairly steady legs yet. God bless those out there like Michael J. Fox and the fighter Mohammad Ali. They will always be great men and great winners.

 6. My last comment on here is this. There has been some news that the drug "Lipitor" for cholesterol has been a contributor to the signs of Parkinson's. So, we must all look into this for sure."

- Theresa (Terry) Tabar from Ocala, Florida, USA

STORIES FROM PARKIES

"I'll just start with a little preamble on my Parkinson's background. Others can compare theirs to mine.

I have been diagnosed with Parkinson's for a little over 11 years. It started with controllable left hand shaking, at first only during cold weather. Later I found my whole left side started to act lazy. I tended to use my right hand/arm for functions instead of using my left.

At dances I noticed my left leg didn't want to move as well as it used to (especially after a couple of drinks). I'd often say that if I had couple of drinks too many I would walk in a circle as if my left foot was nailed to the floor. When I became the slightest bit stressed my left hand and arm would tend to shake.

Now, along with many other symptoms, I find it extremely hard sleeping at night. Everything bothers me, from itchy skin to muscle spasms, mostly my legs. I find myself on the computer most nights 'til morning. I have tried a couple of sleeping pills but they have not helped. I catch up on my rest during the medicated daytime hours.

My present medication is as follows:

Sinemet CR (Levodopa/Carbidopa) 200/50 4 X daily, 4 hrs apart.
Amantadine 100 mg 2 X daily, 8 hrs apart..
Comtan (entacapone) 200mg 3 X daily, 4 hrs apart.
Permax (Pergolide Mesylate) .25 mg 1 X daily, first dosage.

The Permax is slowly being eliminated since I started using the Comtan about 8 weeks ago. It didn't seem to be much help."

- Chris Eggleton from New Brunswick, Canada

"First, about getting a diagnosis. It took about 4 years, and I had several operations (maybe not needed?). Basically I fell into a gap it seemed between ortho doctors, nerve doctors, and pain doctors. We are so divided up medically that a doctor doesn't really know your history or that you're struggled with the same constellation of symptoms over time.

I had carpal tunnel surgery - then an ulnar nerve decompression surgery, in which some of my elbow bone was removed because I essentially couldn't use my left hand. But I also had clumsiness and weakness in my left leg.....

Finally a thoracic surgeon I'd been sent to, because the first operations caused me to have a frozen left shoulder, wanted to operate and remove my first rib through my armpit and I said "no" not 'til we know what my condition is."

These male doctors wrote "after a lengthy examination ......", which meant they had listened for maybe 10 minutes and examined me for 10 to 20 minutes, they'd exceeded the allotted time for me. I could hardly describe the symptoms and the various interventions already tried in short time.

I'd been to some alternative doctors too - deep tissue massage (this really hurt), acupuncture (helped none), chiropracty (no help), and facial massage (you guessed it). Nothing helped the pain in the weak muscles on the left side - mostly in leg and arm and shoulder.

In fact, I stood with my left wrist on my waist because the muscle spasms would pull my arm up like that. And due to my frozen facial expression, people acted as if I didn't hear when they mocked me. My own mother said to a crowd of relatives one Christmas, "look at Terri standing with her arm like this (mimicking me) and I thought, "Does she not know I'm here?"

Finally, a female doctor with her degrees both in Rehabilitation and in Neurology spent 2 1/2 hours with me and stated, "Your problems are not peripheral (arm/leg/shoulder), your problems are central!" I didn't know what that meant at first, but she explained, "Brain, not muscle".

She scheduled me for a brain scan to rule out MS, and I was relieved someone had the big picture maybe, though I was scared to death. In the meantime, I had no one to talk to. Friends had long grown tired of listening, and my relatives didn't believe I really had a problem I couldn't control.

So with that, I was sent to a big hospital an hour and a half away, and there was found to have PD. I was so shocked I argued with the doctors - "No, that's old people- I'm only 45!". After being alone and having cried 40 minutes in the bathroom (partly out of relief to finally know, but terrible fear too) and trying over an hour to find where I'd left my car in the various color zones of this big place, I managed to drive, though not well, home.

It felt like I'd joined someone else's life - someone I didn't know - and had lost my own. I didn't know me with Parkinson's disease! I was confused to the point of real terror and couldn't talk to anyone without crying.

I cried at work too - a relatively new job as a psychologist in a maximum security prison treating chronically mentally ill inmates. The stress made me make small, non clinical mistakes, and my boss always caught these glitches and confronted me and then I cried.

At this time no one could even ask me a general question about how I was without my reacting with copious tears. I wrote poetry and most of it had a suicidal bent, not because that's what I wanted, but because I was thoroughly confused about how to live the life imposed on me by this disease.

After I was fired and surrendered my license to practice, I was really lost and afraid - so afraid! My family continued not to understand nor tolerate my crying. Why couldn't I just cope like everyone else?

So antidepressants were needed to stop the continual tears. Dry-eyed I still did not know what to do. I couldn't support myself as I applied for Disability and could not get unemployment at the same time.

I further discredited myself with my family by trading several cars downwardly as I needed cash; lost my house as I had to turn it over to the bank to avoid bankruptcy, and struggled to help my daughter have any sense of security with me as sick, divorced, fired, without money, and sick. It was truly hell and I wondered if God was punishing me for my mistakes known and unknown. Fear was like an animal always ready to consume me whole.

So I had this life to live. It came time for my daughter's emancipation into college, and yes, she lives with her boyfriend I'm sure generating for herself the family and security she'd needed with me. I'd met someone, who after 2 and 1/2 years with me and my uncertainties, broke up with me "to give me a chance for someone more able" to meet my growing needs, and I was lost again. I just couldn't live a normal life with all the meds I took; the cycles of emotion and physical limitation; and pain; the fear.

The loving folks at church seemed to be able to stick by me no matter what, and even seemed to notice when I did do something well- like write for the newsletter, or speak up in Sunday School class.

I, after years of prayer, met the "good man" I'd begged God for the weekend before the latest chapter of my illness occurred - deep brain stimulation surgery. I'd been referred to a big university hospital at UNC-Chapel Hill, and right off the bat - first visit - I was asked if I'd consider brain surgery. I was shocked, answering "Do I need brain surgery?" The answer made me even more nervous - "You will."

So, this doctor died unexpectedly of heart failure, and I was transferred to my present neurologist. He took over the theme of brain surgery, especially as I was in my 9th year of medication. They had been raised to high doses of "dopamine agonists" known to cause hallucinations from long-time use. And when my medicine didn't work, I was barely able to walk. I had such freezing and shuffling that it could take an eternity to cross a room.

Once at home alone, I failed to reach the toilet 6 feet in front of me and soiled myself profusely. Though I had no witnesses I felt deeply ashamed and again the crying came. Instead of feeling like a sick person, I felt like the most inept person living - couldn't even go to the bathroom on time! The fear returned- what if this had been in public- at church for instance- what was I to do?

The UNC neurologist had the answer- deep brain stimulation surgery. There came a time when my appointment consisted of reading the DBS booklet and having my questions answered. Then there came a day, after many tests to see if I was truly a suitable candidate, when I had to make my own decision whether or not to go forward with the surgery.

What stuck in my mind is what still sticks now - "It's your best shot- you know where it goes from here without surgery, and it's probably your best shot for a normal life."

Well I want to be there when my daughter marries, and play with grandchildren on my knee, and hopefully after they walk, walk with them. So it seemed I made the only decision I had, if I still wanted to live.

I thought I'd been thoroughly prepared for the surgery, but how do you prepare someone to be awake while an electric drill bores into their skull? Or after having to bare it for hours on the one side, having to tolerate a new beginning on the other. Or to live with the wire in my neck and head that's big and thick and uncomfortable. Or the fear when pain did occur.

I was one of the unfortunate recipients of this process or to undergo long hospitalization for meningoencephalitis, herpes/simplex. It started with reoccurring headaches in the months following DBS which would stop me in my tracks and cause me to cry in pain.

I would avoid physical activities when the headaches came, as I feared having something explode in my aching head thus ending my life. My current love would grasp my head and remark on the heat he felt from my incision and the puffiness of my head protrusions (where I have caps to close the burr holes in my skull).

I tried to be alright and visit him in his home country of England 3 months after DBS. We fell in love and wanted to marry and for him to move to the USA, but I needed to see his home and meet his friends and relatives. I knew not to let my body be searched with the magnets at the airport, but I did not know the pain I would encounter on the flight while in the air. My brain seemed to swell until it felt like it was being painfully squeezed by my skull which I feared might spilt open.

After hurting until fear took the upper hand and made me seek help, I walked to the back and whispered to an attendant that I needed to seek medical personnel on the plane. She questioned me further, which just brought on the inevitable crying, and the plane's manager was sought. He finally made an announcement for such persons to come to the back of the plane. I marveled again, as I listened to the announcement, that I was the person causing the problem.

They gave me reassurances, tranquilizers, and pain killers which got me there, though not without causing me to blank out upon landing. I had no idea where my luggage was when my love inquired, and he wondered aloud how I had managed. My eyes were barely open, the gland under my chin on one side of my neck swollen out, and I was unsteady on my feet.

But we made the best of it sightseeing as if things were normal, taking care that I had my pills, until about a week and a half went by and I had a headache I could not ignore. It tore at my skull, so that I blurted into the conversation between my love and his sister that I had to go eat. We were late for dinner and I hoped that would help. It didn't and the next day I backed out of a horseback ride tour of the Moors we had reservations for because I could not imagine putting my pained head aboard the jaunting of a horse.

My love took me straight to a hospital where I entered at 7:30 in the morning with head pain and a 105 degree temperature. I had 4 neurologists but when they agreed they knew not what to do, I was transferred to the Neurology Specialty hospital hours away. And when my spinal fluid was still elevated with white blood cells, I was sent home to America in case the hardware in my head had to come out.

Five days later I was released to come home on a PIC line, which meant I had a tube up my artery into my heart in order for intravenous medication to flow for 2 weeks at home. Now, 5 months after this horrendous experience, during which I hallucinated, became paranoid, and had delusions in the British hospitals away from home, I still marvel that I made it through.

I still have some pain in my head and discomfort with the wires in my neck, but I'm back to the same hope and ambition I had that inspired the positive surgical choice. I want to be there to see my daughter married, I want to have a good long time on earth with my grandkids, and I want to marry this lovely man who helped me through so we can help each other through the rest of life. I want to travel with him, a wish of his, and avoid so much pain or disability that I can't live out my life as normal as possible, as pain free as possible, and as productively as possible.

In 2 weeks I'll attend a reception to display photos from my previous travels, including England, and hope to start a photography business. I get by staying busy with making my dreams come true. I hang onto the support I can get with the people who have made it their business to understand, and don't bother giving explanations to those who haven't.

I get up every morning hopeful of accomplishment and do what I can to enjoy my journey. And I think a lot about the love I can show my daughter, my lover, my friends, and anyone else in this at times scary, lonesome, and painful life we have together on our needy planet. May God care for us all!"

- Terri Johnson

"Parkinson's 101"

"It started with a sore right shoulder which was easily treated with a cortisone shot. A sore shoulder for a second time and a twitch in my right hand and I was off to see the neurologist (Dr. Khamishon).

I was sure it was just a pinched nerve from lifting too many weights. Almost the first thing the doctor asked me do was to walk down a hall as he watched for reasons only he knew. I found out later one of the things he was looking for was if I was swinging each arm when walking normally. A classic sign of Parkinson's is lack of both arms swinging.

Not sure what I was thinking but on future doctor visits when asked again to walk I had both arms swinging like a German storm trooper, high and far! Might have been thinking if I could fool Dr. Khamishon I could fool Parkinson's.

If nothing else I created a little doubt because the doctor tried a few new tests. Touch your toes, stand on one foot, and touch your nose with one finger. Heck, this is nothing more than the drunk driver tests and I've been practicing this test for years! I'd pass easy. No way I'd have Parkinson's.

Then Dr. Khamishon says make both hands like a claw or pincher and open and close each hand as fast as you can. My right hand moved in slow motion compared to the left hand. Busted on a simple open and close your hand test. Damn! Have tried many times since then to speed up my right hand hoping I could take the test again and not have Parkinson's. No Chance."

- Dan Thomas from San Diego, USA

"All of my life I have considered myself a rather private person. Not an introvert, but to myself in many ways. Oddly I went into the retail business and always enjoyed communicating with total strangers as well as "the regulars". Although a private person, I did have a gift to gab.

The business encompassed camera sales, photo finishing and custom framing. I worked 6 days a week (sometimes 7). In my late 20's I wasn't convinced that I

215

felt all that great so I started playing badminton for exercise. In case you are unaware don't be too quick to judge badminton as a "kiddy back yard game". Played correctly and seriously it is similar to tennis but the hardest hit tennis ball may be clocked at maybe 120 mph, whereas the badminton shuttle can be smashed around 140+.

In my very early 40's I was annoyed by that first telltale tremor and I'm sure you know how the following years progressed. Probably the hardest thing I had to do was give up the one sport that enjoyed so much. As well the interaction of the friends and club members. Having that private side to me really brought to the forefront that common companion of parkinson's and that is the "hide-yourself-away" thing that happens.

Other than possibly 3 friends and my wife, it is a VERY rare time that I will discuss it. Who in the world wants to hear someone whining about their aches and pains? Parkinson's being the way it is, I could feel (and look) absolutely terrible for 8 hours and then for 45 minutes, feeling pretty good, venture out into public and invariably someone with the best intentions will say, "You're looking really good". Half an hour later if my door rang, I may not be able even respond.

It's like a roller coaster that no one else is on. It shoots skyward much too fast and then free-falls only to spend about 97% of it's time underground where it's murky, damp and dark. Then it comes out just enough to tease you then back it goes.

WOW....This appears to be the ramblings of a tortured soul now that I look back. However, I will leave it in its disjointed condition.... that's the way it came off of my finger tips.

Just to update you a bit. About 1½ years ago I was accepted for DBS and went ahead with that. There is NO doubt that procedure helps. Sleep is much more pleasant now where before it was just torture. Although there are times it isn't able to do enough, my frustration with its lackluster performance is quickly put to rest by turning the DBS off. Then I am promptly reminded where I would be without it.

You may have noticed the lack of a capitol "p" when I spell parkinson's. That is to demonstrate my total lack of respect that I have for this disease. I have fought it every hour of every day for about 15 years. At times when the anger boils to the surface... and it does, it always amazes me that it feels good to let off some steam and get mad at *it*. Well I can't stay mad all the time, but I still can express the never ending dislike I have for this unwelcome visitor and start *his* name with a capitol is something I can't do.

WOW...........Again, now this appears to be the rantings of a madman.

Actually the feelings I've listed above are negative for the most part there are

216

some good times dispersed here and there as life moves on. They MUST be what one looks forward to.

- Sandy

PS: Hardly a day goes by when I don't think of the exercise, fun, sweat and exhaustion that badminton brought to me. I am very sure that the last 15 years were made easier because of the mental and physical exercise it brought."

"I am now at my home in a retirement village in Florida. I'll be here until May 1st. The village has a good support group for PD. We meet every Thursday from 1:00 to 3:00. There are approx. 30 to 35 people. The first hour is stretching and strengthening, and the second hour is for group discussion.

Our exercise class is conducted by a dynamic 5th grade school teacher from New York whose husband has PD. She is the author of the My Goal mantra. In my opinion, it is a powerful tool which I use every day. Since switching from the YMCA exercise regimen to this stretching and strengthening, I have improved my movement tremendously.

The author of this mantra is Joanna."

My Goal is:

To be as independent and self
reliant as possible, as long as
possible-if not indefinitely.

I will do this through stretching,
strengthening and balancing
exercises and ADL's.
(activities for daily living)

- Vince from Pennsylvania, USA

"Parkinson's Disease and a 'Gift' "

"I was diagnosed at 51 with Parkinson's disease. I remember hearing the diagnosis and crying as my husband's arms encompassed me. But little did I know that along with the diagnosis would come a gift.

After my diagnosis I continued to work but began to feel an urge to create. It began as new product ideas in my job ... where I worked administratively and product development was not part of my responsibility. One idea actually resulted in a product being placed on the market and a submission for a patent in my name.

Although medication helped, the disease progressed and I decided to leave my twenty-three year career. That is when I began to dream books. That's right – I dream the plots of mystery books. I wake up with the plot of an entire novel in my head. In eleven months I wrote an unheard of five manuscripts, and have since completed three more.

At first I wrote manuscripts to share with family and friends, but was encouraged to try publishing my work. To my delight, my first manuscript, "Lessons Learned," was published. My books are murder mysteries with an inspirational flare – what a combination, huh?

Many have theories regarding my "gift," such as: "The healthy portion of the brain is being over-stimulated by the medications;" or "As with someone who loses one of their senses, you've gained something;" and the one I tend to believe, "You've always had the ability and with portions of the brain being affected by PD, other portions of the brain are being used more often and are more pronounced." Doctors do agree on one thing, however - no one knows for sure why this has happened.

I enjoy my new-found writing ability and continue to write. I've also added painting to my list of creative outlets. When my medications are working, I love to paint and have several hanging in my home and some in the homes of friends.

I have recently come upon an Internet site of many others with Parkinson's disease who have discovered new found abilities. Pick up a pencil or a brush and give it a try – maybe you've received a gift too!

In addition to my creative outlets, I found that hard exercise helps me to sustain my flexibility, strength and balance. I work with a trainer three times a week and workout twice a week on my own. Would you know I have Parkinson's disease if you saw me? Maybe. My stride has shortened and I have occasional bouts with tremors on my left side-–but hey, I'm still smiling.

Deal with the cards your dealt. Life is good - make the most of it".

- Janis Anderson Yelton from Villa Hills, Kentucky, USA

"I am 70 this year and weigh 145 pounds. I first became aware that something was going wrong with me around nine years ago when my golf handicap rose from 18 to 28 despite all my efforts. I had lost co-ordination, then the walking problems began, and the tremors on my left side.

One day trying to play golf, a lady remarked to my wife have you seen the chicken man (me). My wife had been telling me to see a doctor for some time, but I did not think for one moment that I was seriously ill. My symptoms were recognized by a person who had a friend with Parkinson's and I was persuaded to see a specialist.

I could not be ill! Me who during my working life hardly ever had a day off . I played football, table tennis to a high standard, ran half marathons, worked out in the gym, did step aerobics, went skiing regularly, and I was careful with my diet. However, I was diagnosed with PD.

Three years ago I moved to South Africa. I play golf three times per week, off a handicap of 20, walking behind my electric cart, winning the odd prize from time to time. Work out in the gym. My current medication is three Carbilev 125 (Sinemet) (sometimes I manage on two) and one Azilect daily."

- Reginald

"On May 20, 1996, my personal physician confirmed that I had PD. She also said I had slight Brady Intestinal, which is minimal cogwheel rigidity of my upper extremities. This includes slight shuffling and slight instability. I was prescribed 5 mg. Eldepryl twice a day.

For the next three years my symptoms were mild. Friends noted changes in my posture, locomotion and facial expression. I was still able to golf, do the necessary yard work, and handle the minor projects within the home. I considered myself fortunate in not having any tremors.

In 2000, 0.25 mg. of Requip three times per day was added to my medication. It caused sleep attacks, and I had to stop taking it. My medication was changed to 200mg. of Sinemet, three times per day replacing both the Requip and Eldepryl. The Sinemet worked fairly well for two years, and in 2002, it was replaced with 150 mg. of Stalevo to give me more "on time". This is the same medication I take today (three times per day).

I failed to mention that since the start of my PD, two thing shave been happening in addition to the other items mentioned above. 1. My writing has become smaller and smaller to the point where I am unable to write at all. It is very difficult to write my name. 2. My speech has deteriorated to the point where I cannot be understood.

My balance problems started in the winter of 2004. While vacationing in Florida, I started falling frequently and I saw a neurologist while there who said that a cane would help. I obtained a cane and used it for six months. My balance problems worsened and the falls increased in severity. The neurologist recommended that I get a walker, so I did in early 2006. I have used the walker for a year and now have a powered wheelchair.

Well, that wraps up my ten year Parkinson's experience. Now, I will try to answer some of your questions. I was never interested deep brain simulation {DBS} since I never had the tremors. Some of the fellows I knew from the Parkinson support group. One was a complete success, and his tremors were eliminated. The second one did not do as well.

There are several things I would highly recommend for the Parkinson's patient to do. One is he or she should join a Parkinson's support group as soon as they are told that they have PD. It certainly does wonders for your moral. You get to meet people who are facing the same problems as you.

They meet once a week and the cost is free. The meeting lasts about two hours. The first part of the meeting is an open discussion where any new Parkinson information is discussed. The second part is devoted to exercises that help the Parkinson patient.

After exercising you have a 15 minute relaxing period where soft soothing music is played while the instructor reads comforting words. Also they have a general luncheon where other support groups are invited. They also have a speaker that is extremely knowledgeable about Parkinson's.

The other item that is very important to the patient is therapy and proper exercise."

- John M. Desimone

"I don't have much to say. Going downhill fast and have trouble typing. I still don't have the shakes but all else is wrong. Falling frequently and they tried balance therapy. Did a lot of downhill skiing and I was holding my legs too close. However I did learn when skiing to roll when you are falling and I have never been hurt bad.

Trouble swallowing pills and eating so they taught me to take small bites and thicken water when swallowing pills using Speech Therapy. Diabetic 2 so I take pills and have special shoes. Trouble urinating so I got a rotor rooter and they took out cancer and I still have problems.

Still have sense of humor and hopes are high. They want me to talk and move slow and it is hard for wife to realize this. Oh, to top it off I have double vision which is corrected by many pair of glasses. Sorry I could not give you a better outlook but I do exercise with a group, 3 times weekly and there are people in worse shape."

- Jerry

"I have only known I've had Parkinson's for 2 years and six months and have only just started using email. I am 61 years old and have had some problems with medication.

The one wonderful thing for me is the support and genuine caring of my group of friends, all retired teachers. We meet for lunch monthly and they always ensure I am collected and returned home safely. I also go out every Saturday to the movies or coffee with a special friend. By keeping social contact and making the most of every day, I feel I cope better with my Parkinson's. Having a wonderful husband caring for me makes me feel very blessed."

- Lyn. Armidale

"I was diagnosed over three years ago, and even though I was given an MRI, I remained in denial and with one symptom, tremor in my left hand, I felt the neurologist was mistaken. One and a half years later I made an appointment with a second neurologist with Baylor in the medical center. I liked her very much and when she confirmed my Parkinson's, I accepted her diagnosis.

She offered me an opportunity to participate in a study the clinic was starting to test Rasagiline. Each month I am tested by her and a group of nurses. Blood pressure, urine analysis, melanoma, my walking, tremor and balance. I feel I am doing very well.

I am upbeat and positive, enjoy going there and submit to a phone question and answer for their study, in which all my answers have been in the negative. In other words, no symptoms that they ask for (ex. need help dressing, miss any work or activities etc.).

Although I believe my symptoms reveal a very slow progression in my disease, mostly I don't dwell on it. When the tremor comes and goes, it does not seem to interfere with any activities I pursue.

If there is one thing I believe helps me, it would have to be a daily exercise program which includes a daily swim and water aerobics combination, mostly weekdays in a heated but outdoor pool (which is in our condo complex). I do a half hour walk weekdays, and a two mile walk Sat. and Sun., 1 mile to Starbucks for coffee and then 1 mile back home.

One of the reasons I exercise is because I had a knee replacement 1 1/2 years ago, and my orthopedist recommended swimming over step aerobics I had previously done. So I naturally kept it up. It is something I love to do, and don't need any motivation to continue.

I feel healthy, I am not sure if that's due to the Rasagiline which I took for the first half of the program, or am taking now. I have not noticed any difference. Perhaps in other participants, they may find a difference.

One more thing, I am 73 years old and perhaps getting the disease so has made a difference to the severity, I don't know. I have survived colon cancer which thankfully diagnosed in a relatively early stage, where it had not spread to the tissues. My oncologist said I am now cancer free. I feel very lucky, really."

- Maureen

"I was diagnosed with Parkinson's over 16 years ago. I am 74. I am still receiving an income as a sales agent, although I do not do a lot of work. I attend the movement clinic at Toronto Western hospital. I am under Dr Tony Lang's care.

This is a teaching hospital and I am first screened by doctors in training to be movement specialists. They give me a complete work-up every six months. For some reason I always show my very best side during the examination. One doctor from Boston told me that I was the best condition of anyone with having had it for so long.

My wife died in April 2003. My very stable condition has begun to slide. I have managed to play golf four times per week but last summer I was getting dyskinesia. The golf became too much for me. I have been going to an acupuncturist for two years. I am influenced by him. He suggested I reduce my medication over time at least 10 weeks. He advised against taking Mirapex Requip. My Parkinson's has also been in my legs. I suffer from numbness in my left leg.

I was encouraged to go back to sing with a large welsh choir. We performed in the Albert Hall amassed choir of 1000 voices and did four other small concerts in Wales.

I had contracted walking pneumonia 2 days before leaving for England. I was in bad shape but the other choir members are very supportive and took great care of me.

Two days before I went for my work-up in August 2006, I was having a lot of trouble with dyskinesia. I called a friend of mine who has Parkinson's and he told me that he had added Amantadine to his diet of pills. Dr. Lang had prescribed Amantadine. The day before my work up I took one Amantadine. It seemed to help. I took two on the day of my work-up and when I got there I performed like a trained seal.

I told Dr. Lang what I had done and I am now taking 3 per day along with 4 X 1/2 Levodopa 100/25. It makes quite a difference but I think that it might be affecting me emotionally. I'm not my usual gregarious self. I believe that you should try to keep your pills to a minimum."

- Anonymous

"If I give you a few facts about myself it might help you to see the problem from my perspective. I am now 71 years old, 6 ft tall and slightly overweight at about 210/220 pounds, I have always been reasonably active.

I first learned that I had Parkinson's about 2 and a half years ago when I began to notice the tremor in my left hand whilst driving (I am right handed by the way, which makes life a little easier).

Further ways PD has manifested itself are in a slower gait, and shorter steps, but I am not shuffling. I am uncertain of my balance because I am always looking down to see what I might trip over. This contributes to a slight stooping of my shoulders.

My specialist and his nurse (who is marvelous and in my opinion could do the doctors work) have both commented verbally and in writing that my attitude will see me through.

I have a positive acceptance of the PD in as much as I am trying very hard not to let it inhibit the things I do. It's difficult at times but I am endeavoring to carry on my life as it was before I was diagnosed. I still walk my dog for about 90 minutes each morning in the local woods, come rain or shine, I still go 10 pin bowling, although I have cut this down to once a week.

Because of the balance problems my handicap has suffered, and I get little exasperated, but mostly I still enjoy it. I still do my DIY, but the fiddly bits suffer a little and would you believe I am in the second term at adult education classes of a calligraphy course. That also could be better, but I find it wonderfully therapeutic.

When I was first diagnosed the specialist told me not to worry. I can remember asking if it was painful and if it was terminal. Getting negatives I responded with "In that case I shan't worry too much". I try to keep that frame of mind when friends inquire. I attempt to inject a little levity into the situation by telling them how awkward it is to eat peas and tell them that I have had to give up the bomb disposal work.

Basically what I am saying I suppose is that by keeping a positive mood and not letting "the monkey on my back" stop me doing the things I want to do, I can lead a reasonable, if at times exasperating and irksome life.

I don't know if you have ever read a cartoon strip called "Calvin and Hobbes", I am sure that it came here from the states. One little saying that cropped up was **"THINK POSITIVE"**.

Hope this helps."

- George

"In September 2005 I began attending a Parkinson's support group in my area, having been diagnosed about 5 months earlier with PD. I noticed another first-time attendee, a gentleman wearing a big hat and carrying a big walking stick. I think we sat near one another and conversed for a short time.

Over the next several monthly meetings we'd talk briefly, and at one point ran into one another at a local thrift store and he didn't seem to place where we'd met, though we conversed at some length.

In the spring a member of our group committed suicide and the rest of us decided to stay in better contact between meetings.

In June my doctor changed my meds, leaving me with a substantial supply of unused pills of the old kind. I offered them to the group as some have a hard time paying for meds. My friend accepted the offer and dropped by my home to obtain them. As a thank-you he returned on another day to chop and stack firewood for me.

We found we enjoyed visiting and had much in common. After helping him through a medical emergency in July we drew even closer. He's 74, I'm 66 and we decided we wanted to spend the rest of our lives together and didn't have 50 years to spend on a long courtship so were married in August after counseling by his pastor. We honeymooned in September with my church's family camping trip.

We decided to live in my home, now ours, and sell his. Our biggest challenge is reducing our belongings in order to fit them in.... we have no regrets six months later and are having the time of our lives. Each day is better than the day before.... We both feel that if Parkinson's was the price for getting to know one another it was worth it."

- April and Bob

"I've learned not to multi task as much as I used to. When I had to leave the high school classroom as a teacher I knew that I had to fill my day with something.

I started working on my fabric stash creating whatever I could think of. It has been relaxing and rewarding. I also renewed my interest in stamped cross stitch. I could only do it a maximum of 30 minutes at a time (sometimes 15 min.) but it was excellent therapy for my hands and sitting in bed relaxed me before going to sleep. It has been rewarding to see the accomplishments.

I have learned to leave my disease in God's hands and to not feel sorry for myself (most of the time). I spend quite a bit of time studying the Bible. That has helped to keep my mind active. I plan to study more Spanish when I get tired of sewing. I have a Masters degree in Spanish and don't want to lose my fluency and reading ability in it.
I am fortunate so far to be on the same dosage of medicine now for 2 years."

- Phyllis

"I was 34 years old when I noticed my right hand Index finger began the movement that was eventually diagnosed as the dreaded monster (Parkinson's disease). The finger would just continue to "drum" uncontrollably all the time. I could make it stop if I concentrated on nothing else but the finger. As soon as the concentration broke it would start again.

After a year or so the drumming turned into a shaking and by then it was the entire hand and lower arm. At this time I was employed with a Sheriff's Dept. I was a Lieutenant over several deputies, as well as jail administrator. The shaking of my hand had gotten to the point that it had become embarrassing therefore I would keep my hand in my pocket or sit on it when sitting, always trying to hide it.

It took it seven years to get take over the entire right side of my body. On my own I decided not to pursue my career of choice any longer therefore leaving it behind. I went to several doctors and they all diagnosed me with the same results. All ways thinking I was to young to have this happen to me, I finally accepted the diagnoses.

At the time i was a single dad of two great God sent gifts a daughter Marissa and A son Sam. I shared with them what I was facing and not knowing much of the disease, just told them that we had to continue sticking together as a family and in prayer. My kids have been very inspirational and know when I am having a bad day. At times like this, without being asked they step up and help me and take care of me. during "off periods" they ask if I have taken my medications.

On October of 2004 I went through Deep Brain Stimulation surgery on the left brain to control the tremors and rigidness on right side my body. by now my entire right side shook uncontrollably. I could no longer hide it. At times I was embarrassed to go anywhere, thinking my kids would be embarrassed, to my surprise they told me that they were not embarrassed when they were out in public with me.

After DBS in 2004 I noticed no slowing down on the advancement of the disease. Two years later my left side fell victim to the "monster. By this time simple task had become chores that required lots of concentration. Getting dressed was a big chore when I used to get dressed in five minutes now was taking me up to thirty minutes. Buttoning up a shirt tying my shoes brushing my teeth and even holding a fork or spoon had become difficult.

In September 2006 I went and had DBS done on the right brain to control problems on left body. In January of 2007 I went to the hospital to have the electrodes re-set. This was done because I had taken a pretty hard fall on my head two months after the surgery. And as a result probably "jarred" the electrodes or caused some damage to them let alone my head.

After that fall, the right stimulator did not function as well as before therefore resulting in yet another entrance into the head. After a month went by I went to the neurosurgeon for a post-op, and adjustment. The doctor and his assistant both tried several combinations to try and help me get rid of the tremors and rigidness. Well my body never responded to the several combinations.

By this time I was beginning to experience problems with swallowing, and more frequent problems with balance. There were days I could speak clearly and days that I had to really concentrate on what I wanted to say and make sure it come out.

Two or three days prior to going to the doctors' I had not been able to speak and if I did it sounded very slurred, low tone and slow. On the day of the visit I was so excited because I was going for an adjustment and those were always good. I could also talk loud and clear.

Well on the way home it was the total opposite, I was very upset and could care less if I could speak or not because I did not want to share the results of the visit with anyone. I had just been dealt a hand that I couldn't win with. All along the doctor had made the remark that my progression was advancing too fast. Well after the no response on the DBS I was told that he suspected that I had gone into Parkinson's Plus. And we all know the end results there.

I'm only 42 years old and think it's not fair, but I think it has and will continue making me a stronger person. I no longer sit and dwell on the condition; instead I want to live not just be alive. I try and enjoy my children more and actually listen to them. They are aware of what the road ahead holds and are very supportive. Everyday I thank the good Lord for allowing me to see a new sunrise (one of my pleasures) and the strength and privilege to be with my kids one more day.

I continue to work, because I do not want to give into this Monster more than he/she has already taken. Some days it is with great difficulty just to get up and go to work. But I will not give up. Not in my vocabulary.

My advice to people with PD is just think there are people in this world with more serious illnesses, so keep your chin up and continue your journey. Suck it up and cowboy up."

- James Melendez, Texas

"It's all about attitude. When I finally got through Mirapex and Requip and started taking Sinemet, I was faced with canceling a long awaited trip to Costa Rica. I decided to go anyway and here's what happened.

One of our excursions was to visit Rara Avis, an ecological paradise at the top of a mountain. Access was through a three hour ride with a four wheel drive tractor pulling a wagon up the hill. As it turned out the tractor was broken at the top of the mountain. The alternative was to ride horses for about two hours and then walk "for a while" the rest of the way.

Being in a rainforest, naturally the downpour began. When we reached the halfway house, two young volunteers met us for the "hike". We tromped straight uphill through three foot deep tractor ruts in the rain and mud. Fortunately I found a walking stick and after a couple of slippery hours made it to the top. It was then that I decided that you can if you think you can and it's made all the difference for me. I still have that stick today."

- Mike

"I was shocked the first time I was told I had Parkinson's but I carried on with life. I try to forget about it. It is hard though when I can't do things I used to be able to or they take twice as long.

My best advice to all that have this disease is to carry on. The best thing I find that helps a lot Sunday mornings is when my mate takes me around to the club for a beer or two.

I see my mates and after two hours all I can say after seeing them is that a laugh and a smile are far better than medication. This is what I find helps in my life As we say in England, a laugh and a smile a day helps you rest and play.

I hope I have helped in some way. Keep smiling. Get on with life. We still have something to give."

- Jim from England

"I find life to be so interesting in how things come back to you.....

A few years ago when my children were young I home schooled them. On an educational standpoint I'm sure this was a mistake. But life is made up of more than that. Education is vital, yes. But there must be balance.

For example: Doctors are expected to obtain so much information and peoples' lives hang on the decisions they make. Wow, nerve wracking for sure. But what about the emotional factor?

Recognize that these issues hold a huge emotional side as well. To find a doctor who has both sides of this type of care is extraordinary! So I figure if I did nothing at the very least I taught matters of the heart.

Part of my teaching included a community service. So we pondered awhile and decided on MIFA. At that time the Collierville Library was looking for volunteers to come serve lunch to a small group of elderly people and play bingo as well. Perfect! So we decided to dedicate every Tuesday to that.

They were a great group of people. All ladies and one gentleman. Oh how they enjoyed my boys. The ladies were talkative and at times sassy even. And the man was quiet and gentle. You could feel his spirit and his eyes were so kind. His name was Mr. Grady.

He struggled to walk and do some of the simple things we all take for granted. But never did he give up or become frustrated. Pride with grace. He at times would ask for assistance which I was always thrilled to help. Despite his physical needs his mind was sharp and he loved to play dominos.

He was a natural wiz with numbers. And was so very patient with my boys and enjoyed teaching them how to play. We loved him dearly.

Although he thought our only lesson was how to play dominoes, we know and still talk about his amazing strength despite adversity.

One day I asked Mr. Grady what his condition was exactly. He told me Parkinson's. I truly never gave it another thought because he was NOT his disease! He was Mr. Grady! A very sweet yet strong man who had so very much to offer all those he came into contact with.

228

Over time I have thought back on those days and how glad I am that my boys got to experience this. Now those of you who know me are thinking wow how ironic! Yes it is! My lesson was so much bigger than I could have ever imagined. And when I have days were I struggle and I begin to get frustrated with my disease, I think about my dear friend Mr. Grady and how Parkinson's was just a small part of who he was.

We all possess the ability to do great and wonderful things. But it's our perception of great and wonderful that holds us back. No I can't physically go and build a house for the less fortunate. Or become a nurse and care for those in need. But I can smile and take time to listen. I can offer all that I am with love in my heart. And I can show how to have joy amongst the burdens. Not to mention I can play a mean game of dominos....

Isn't it funny how life has a way of coming back to you full circle?"

- Paula Lyon

"At the end of 2003 I retired as a "Front line" Police officer (Sgt. Rank) with 31 years service. I went straight into a civilian police role in criminal investigations. During the last year of my service I injured my left shoulder which led to restricted mobility in that area.

In 2004 I decided to have this investigated by MRI full body scan. It didn't explain the shoulder problem, but led to discovery I had osteoporosis, hiatus hernia and a liver problem, which was wrongly diagnosed as cancer of the liver, by a specialist.

Eight weeks later it was found to be "Water cysts" on the liver. I started to suffer from left arm tremors and dragging left leg. You guessed it, Parkinson's was diagnosed. In the same year, diagnosis also confirmed Cervical dystonia (Torticollis). I have now been recently diagnosed with Diverticular disease.

As a young boy, I always had a healthy diet, loved fruit, vegetables and whole meal bread. I also kept pretty fit up to my retirement. In my opinion and from research I have read, I believe the illnesses are all related. I also believe the trauma and stress suffered from being a police officer and my sad divorce led to my brain giving up to Parkinson's. I hope one day the "Cosmic Cavalry" will come to my rescue!

Despite above, I live an independent life, full time shift working occupation and I also look after my elderly mother. My long term girlfriend has recently ended our relationship, which really hurts.

I keep going by stoic determination, that one day a cure will be found. My daily living is helped by regular physical exercise, body massage and maintenance by a specialist physiotherapist."

- John from United Kingdom

"My PD Story"

"As with many of us it is my mother who has been diagnosed with PD. I'll do my best to write this as a text rather than a biography to better help those who are in search of answers.

Mom called me one day stating that she wasn't feeling well and hadn't felt well for a few weeks and wanted me to take her to her PCP. She made an appointment and she got in that same day. Her blood pressure was sky high and she described many symptoms-blurred vision, numbness in her legs from the knee down, tremors in her left hand and arm, nausea and dizziness. Also, the sensation of a spider web on her left cheek was another symptom.

The doctor was nice and told her to increase her blood pressure medicine, gave her a referral to a neurologist and sent her home to wait the ten days to see the specialist. He talked briefly about the tremor but never mentioned PD.

In a short time the tremors became worse causing violent shaking of the left arm and eventually the entire left side of her body. She has a pace maker and she insisted that it was causing all of her symptoms but she had just seen the pacer technician and he said that it was functioning properly. So we went to her cardiologist and he in turn said that all was in order and to go and see the neurologist as scheduled.

She became even worse so we spent an entire day in the emergency room at a regional hospital where many tests were made, even a CT of her brain and neck. All the tests came back negative. During the ER visit her blood pressure and heart rate went so high during one of her shaking episodes that the machine sounded off an alarm. I thought that now they will do something. No, the nurse came in reset the machine and said that there was an "error"! The ER doctor said that there was no emergency so he could not admit her. By now she was showing sighs of the "mask". The left side of her face was drooping slightly.

We drove home knowing that although they had found nothing wrong there was something terribly wrong. We did begin to speak of PD as someone we knew had it. My grandmother on my father's side of the family. But still I did not have enough information to make that call and the doctors were not saying any such thing.

All symptoms continued to get worse. She complained of a shaking feeling in her stomach. She wanted to take her head off and set it to one side. She begged me for Valium, literally, anything to ease her suffering.

By then she had become extremely fearful and anxious. Not one doctor or nurse had mentioned PD to us. It was dreadful to say the least. By the time we were able to see the neurologist she could not walk alone, she could not fasten her own clothes or put on her own shoes. She could not put her own feet into the car without assistance. New symptoms appeared over night. It was like a runaway train, there was no stopping it!

The neurologist asked questions and watched her movements. He confidently said that she has PD and prescribed Reequip. I was relieved to have a diagnosis but mom was devastated. She broke down. He told her that it was treatable and gave us some samples to get her started. It was like a miracle. Within minutes of the first dose she felt better, better enough to stop at a restaurant for lunch before going home.

I was exhausted from several weeks of care giving and research seeking help nutritionally and homeopathically. I also have a job and a family and I live in another town, which is 45 minutes away. Two of my siblings offered to stay with mom over the weekend so that I could rest. I was in great need of rest. I was drained emotionally, physically and mentally.

By Monday morning when I returned to my position as caregiver I was amazed at mom's recovery! She was her pre-PD self again. She had come back to life before my very eyes. I was so very thankful indeed.

However, this was short lived because during my absence my siblings had decided and had convinced my mom that she did not have PD, hat the medication was poison and that she did not need it and they discarded it. Neither one of them had seen mom at her worst. They had only the information which I myself had given them.

How could they not believe me? Why would anyone make up something of that nature? They did not see it for themselves and therefore "denial" became an issue for all of us. I knew that they wanted to stop her diuretic medication and blood pressure medication because my sister had called me about that and I told her to reduce the blood pressure medication but not to stop it. The doctor should be consulted before stopping any medication.

Anyway they had a party for mom over that weekend and she appeared to be all better. Everyone was happy. However, after they left on Monday and the party was over and mom was alone again her symptoms began to reappear. I called the doctor and he called in another prescription for us. I picked it up the same day. She had been off the medication for 3 days.

There was a tug of war between my siblings and myself, which was affecting mom adversely. I totally left it up to mom if she wanted to take the Reequip telling her that at least it was available to her if she needed it. Then it occurred to me to hide it in case my brother decided to discard it again. She actually said to me that she could take it and he would not have to know, she just would not tell him. So she did and felt immediately better.

As time went on she stopped and started taking the medication so many times that I lost count. I totally had to step aside and give her medical care and counsel over to my brother because I felt that he had to be forced to go with her to the doctors. He had to hear their professional advice for himself, as he did not accept it second hand from me.

Also, mom was faced with not knowing what to do or who to believe - me and the doctors or my brother. He did go with her and he simply told the doctors that she did not have PD and their medication was poison and she would not be taking it. He has also told the cardiologist the same thing and she no longer takes her heart medications.

Although she has stopped all medications which were blamed for her symptoms, she continues to have mild symptoms of PD. My brother tells everyone that she does not have PD and never did.

I found Lianna Marie's book after I gave up my position as caregiver to my mom. It cleared up so many questions for me. After reading it I realized that mom has had mild symptoms of PD for several years.

A severe emotional shock triggered the episode with full-blown symptoms. Because my siblings bring great "joy" to my mom she had "on time" when they were with her so they saw her at her best. I saw her at her worst. I did not have the time or the good sense to videotape her episodes. It could have made a difference. The Reequip got her over the hump and allowed her to rest and get back to her right mind. I know that it helped and she would not have survived without it.

My siblings and my mom continue to deny the diagnosis, and in so doing, deny her the proper treatment, which could slow the progress and severity of this disease.

It makes mom happy to be medication free. That in itself is good for her moral, which in turn is good for her PD. She is 78 years old and continues to deny all and blame all on anything and everything from coffee flavoring in her yogurt to her pacemaker. If her symptoms never again progress then we are home free. I pray that they do not.

My advice to you is to do anything and everything that lifts the spirit and cheers the one who suffers from this disease. Nutrition is extremely important and a happy heart is a healing force. Never blame yourself and leave no stone unturned.

Take care of your own needs first or you will be no good to the one who needs your support and help. It is very easy to let your own needs suffer when someone you love and care about needs your help.

I say a prayer for each and everyone who reads this, as I know that you too are reaching out and are in need of answers. May God guide you and light your way. Amen."

- "Z' from Arizona, USA

"I am a retired guidance counselor and was diagnosed with Parkinson's in 2005, when I was 54 years old. I do not have severe symptoms, but the tremor in my right hand and both feet & legs is certainly more than a nuisance.

I have experienced balance problems, staggering, memory loss, and difficulty finding the correct word to use. My neurologist has tried numerous medications (with many unpleasant side effects) and I am now taking only Mirapex and Stalevo. This combination of meds has been the most beneficial. My tremor is controlled most of the time, with most people not noticing it at all.

For balance and muscle strength, I joined the YMCA and take yoga classes 3 times a week - this has helped my balance and stability enormously! I also do the weight machines for strengthening my muscles - I believe just keeping oneself generally healthy will make any disease, including Parkinson's, more tolerable.

I also started taking piano lessons last year (stimulates my mind and eye/hand/mind coordination). I'll never be a concert pianist, but I hope to be able to play a few Christmas carols one day! I attend Bible studies, deliver Meals-on-Wheels, take line-dancing classes and am open to any new adventure that will stimulate me mentally, physically, or spiritually.

I am determined to not let PD ruin my life's activities completely; when I reach a point where I have to give up one thing, I plan to replace it with another that I can do!

Tips:

1. When I got to the point where I could not put on my eye make-up due to my shaky hand, I had permanent eye liner and eyebrows tattooed on (now I am a very conservative person and this was a step way out of my comfort zone). I am SO happy I had this done, it makes me feel better about myself when I feel I look as good as I can. It also means I spend much less time putting on my makeup everyday. It was a little costly, but I saved for it and felt it was a worthwhile

expenditure!

2. I started using an electric toothbrush when brushing with my regular toothbrush became so difficult. This was great - keeps me from getting so frustrated first thing in the morning!

3. I give thanks to God daily that I do not have something worse - like diabetes (which my best friend has) or MS or other debilitating conditions! I am blessed and I believe my spiritual health has a direct effect on my physical & mental health!

4. I try to keep a good sense of humor about PD. I will joke about my shaking and that puts others at ease. Most PD patients I have met do seem to enjoy humor.

5. I keep myself updated on PD research and attend a regular PD support group - this has been invaluable!

- Vennie Evans from Palmyra, Tennessee, USA

"What is this I'm feeling? Trying desperately to keep it all together. Yearning for some control. Yet robbed of my dignity. The very things that come natural to most is turmoil for me. I want to laugh it off. I want to pretend it doesn't exist within me. Do I even remember the day when I had the freedom of thought and movement? No, I don't dare go there. To ponder these things would only cause heartache. For this is my reality now.

They say serious yes, but it won't kill you. Then why does it feel like a slow death? I fear the day that I can no longer connect. The day when I am trapped within my thoughts.

Think of it like this. You are a supervisor of 3 people. You need a very simple task done. You look at them and give them exact directions. You wait. They just stare at you. You can see they want to please you and complete the simple task ahead. Yet they don't understand your directions. So you try again and again.

Now you begin to get angry and frustrated. It can't be your directions for they are correct. You have seen them work for others time and time again. Why is it so difficult now? You want to tell them to forget it you will do it yourself. But you can not. It takes a team to accomplish the task at hand.

Oh God the frustration! You begin to look around. Everyone has not only completed their task but has stopped to see what is wrong with you. Hence the question. What is this I am feeling?

So many emotions...anger, frustration, embarrassment, sadness, and many more.

234

How do I keep my dignity here? The worse part is there are no days off! Everyday you must repeat the same task with the same people. You are trapped in a nightmare.

Some days are better than others. And at times others come to help you. You swallow your pride and graciously except the help. Only to have it start all over again...."

- Paula Lyon

"Why Not Me?"

"The doctor, a slim and authorative man, in his mid forties, got up from his chair and went to his desk and took out a small tool, like a hammer. He returned to where I was sitting and started to check my reflexes by hitting just below my knee and then my arms.

He then checked my arms and legs for rigidity. He asked me to write a sentence on the pad that he gave me. I started out okay but half way through it my writing became very tiny and was not recognizable by the end of the sentence. He asked me if I was able to close and open the buttons of my shirt. I told him that I struggle with them lately. In fact another part of my diagnosis was when the Dr asked me; "Do you enjoy life and can you smile. I told him that "I cannot smile and do not enjoy life much anymore".

This was the big clue that helped with my diagnosis. He returned to his chair and after a short pause he looked at Celia and then he looked at me and said: "At last I have an answer and I am 99% certain. Ned has Parkinson's disease and may have had it for over a year."
My response was silence and shock. I looked at Celia and she too was speechless. We just sat there looking at each other and wondering what the news from the doctor meant.

Was this what we wanted to hear or were we just dreaming or had we heard him correctly? I was in total denial. Was the verdict true? Fear, frustration, even some anger is the emotions that I experienced at this moment. The stages of grief: denial, anger, bargaining etc that I had often used from Dr. Kubler Ross came to mind and I wondered how long it would be before the fifth stage, acceptance. Then I remembered the advice I had shared so often with other people, now I have to work through each stage, one at a time. Yes one stage at a time.

Celia finally broke the silence and asked how sure he was of Parkinson's disease and what in fact did this mean for Ned. He had said: "I am almost 100% sure it is Parkinson's". Would he be able to function normally? How far advanced was the disease? Does it fit some of the symptoms that we just talked about?"

The doctor carried out some more tests and asked some more questions. He then said; "I can start the Parkinson's medicine today and if he has a positive reaction then we know it is Parkinson's. We can treat it with Sinemet, the best medicine we have on the market. This is a powerful drug and works real well. I will start the medication this date."

I am still sitting there in shock and denial, wondering what was in store with this diagnosis and thinking to myself: "Why me? What else do I need?" The doctor noticed my anxiety and looked in my direction and said; "Well Ned the good news is we have come up with a diagnosis and we can treat this disease. I will refer you to a very good Neurologist in Fort Worth, her name is ..."

Three weeks later Celia and I were sitting in her office wondering if she would agree with the above diagnosis and confirm the fact that I had Parkinson's disease. As she entered the small waiting room she looked at Celia and said: "I never know who to expect in my office." She knew Celia from the hospital and she smiled as she looked at me and somehow assured me that I was in the right place.

After a series of more tests she asked me to walk down the hall as she observed my walk.   She checked the rigidity in my limbs and asked me to close my eyes as I stretched out my two hands in front of me. She finally spoke the inevitable words. Perhaps the words that was now all too familiar. "You have Parkinson's disease and may have had it for sometime - maybe a year or more. You are very young to have this disease but look at Michael J Fox, he is younger."

She invited Celia and me across the hall to her office and she explained a little more about the disease and the options for treatment.

Parkinson's is an old disease named after the English Dr. James Parkinson who worked with the disease in 1817. The term "parkinsonism" refers to any condition that involves a combination of the types of changes in movement seen in Parkinson's disease, which happens to be the most common condition causing this group of symptoms.

PD is a degenerative disease of the nervous system associated with trembling of the arms and legs, stiffness and rigidity of the muscles and slowness of the movement (bradykinesia).

I could identify with most of these symptoms and it was finally making a lot of sense. Hence the lack of control of certain movements and trembling. The doctor said that a third of the people affected with P.D. go on to develop senile dementia and seriously affected people may suffer from complications of a stroke.

There is no one cause for Parkinson's. PD is caused by the progressive loss of brain cells (neurons) in the part of the brain called the substantia nigra which produces dopamine. As the cells die, less dopamine is produced and transported to the striatum, the area of the brain that coordinates movement.

The exact reason that the cells of the brain deteriorate is unknown. The disorder may affect one or both sides of the body. With me it was my right side.

She used a simple chart to illustrate what she was saying. Symptoms develop as neurons die off and dopamine levels drop. She said research suggests Parkinson's sufferers may lack other brain chemicals including serotonin (linked to mood).

The doctor said that some people with PD become severely depressed and this happened to me. For almost one year I was being treated for depression with several different medications that were not helping me at all.

She went on to say that PD affects two people in every 1,000 and I am one of that percent. Most patients are over 40 and PD is one of the most common neurological disorders of the elderly.

In a small number of people PD may be inherited. These patients usually develop the disease under the age of 50. Two genes called alpha-synuchlein parakin have been linked to the disease, although others may also be involved. Their exact function is unknown and currently genetic tests for them are not routine, as most data remains experimental.

The common symptoms are tremors, usually while resting, stiffness and muscle cramps known as rigidity, particularly affecting the arms, legs and neck. Slowness in initiating movement known as bradykinesia is also a symptom, along with poor balance and unstable walking. The one that I can identify with is the expressionless face.

In every story there is an angel who plays an important part and my story is no different. The angel in my life is Celia. She was there when I was diagnosed, and she came to the first visit to the neurologist, and many more times since then. She picks up my prescriptions as well as keeping me on track with the many medications.

She is my guardian angel and is always there to keep up my optimism, and always has a supportive and encouraging message for me. There are many times when I feel down and get very frustrated when I cannot do the simple tasks that I was so comfortable with before the onset of Parkinson's.

So often these are the very simple things that we take for granted in everyday living. Something as simple as getting my wallet out of my back pocket, closing a button on my shirt, and numerous other things that were routine for many years.

In all these situations and when I am frustrated with something, Celia is always there to comfort me with a hug and an appropriate word of encouragement. I do appreciate my bride, the one and only love of my life. She is my guardian angel who is always there to help and when my neck aches or my legs are hurting she gives me the strength and motivation to get moving.

She has helped me to turn that original question from 'Why me" to "Why not me". She helped me to appreciate all that I have been given freely every day of my life. I know I have been bestowed many blessings, Michael J Fox called himself "Lucky man," and I too feel lucky and blessed that I can continue to work and drive my truck and do some carpentry work that I love and want to continue to do.

Barbara Thompson the English saxophonist and composer says of her life since her diagnosis; "Although I have Parkinson's and the problems that go with it, it is not the main thing in my life and I am very much getting on with my musical career." I know there are many more people who have accepted the disease of Parkinson.

No two people with PD are exactly the same and each will have a different combination of symptoms. Drug treatment is prescribed to suit the individual, both in terms of dosage and the times the drugs are taken. Each person reacts to his or her drugs in different ways.

To determine how much and what kind of PD medicine will be established by a process of trial and error, and even then may remain optimal for a relatively short period of time because of the progressive nature of the condition.

There is no cure as yet for PD; drugs are used to try to control the symptoms. There are no perfect drugs although there are many promising developments. What the drugs do for PD is to increase the level of dopamine that reaches the brain, stimulate the parts of the brain where dopamine works, or the drugs block the action of other chemicals that affect dopamine.

One of the secrets is to have early diagnosis and there is a good chance of controlling PD and with anti-Parkinson medicine a better quality of life can be maintained for a long time. When somebody has mild symptoms they may decide with their GP to postpone drug treatment until symptoms increase and instead rely on a healthier lifestyle, focusing on exercise, relaxation and diet. And so I conclude with: "Why not me?"

When I was growing up, my neighbor was Ger Maher who was a Philosopher in his own field. He had many insights into life and a favorite saying of his was: "Everybody's shoe pinches somewhere."

- Ned Byrne

STORIES FROM CAREGIVERS

"The greatest challenge I have had as caregiver is the fact that I was pretty much prepared for his becoming more and more dependent on me as far as his physical condition worsened, but was not prepared and had not been told before that the Parkinson's and the medicine could cause hallucinations. That has been his problem also, because he is constantly seeing things and people that are real to him but that I do not see. I hope others may have some ideas to help this."

- Marge from North Carolina, USA

"I find there's a lot to do for someone with Parkinson's. It is very hard to know what to cook for someone like this, as protein seems to make it worse with the medicine when taken 1 1/2 hrs before. This makes my husband freeze up. He has frozen up when he has gone to the store and people in the store had to put him in an electric wheelchair and bring him to his car. At least he does not have a problem driving yet.

I am going to suggest a light weight wheelchair to carry so when this happens I will be prepared. I really cannot help Tom when he gets this way as he is heavy and he says he don't want to hurt me. I'm under a doctors' care as well.

I am not sure what stage Tom might be in. His foot turns in and all his toes go under and the leg is so stiff that he can't bend it. It is painful. His right hand shakes a lot even when he takes the medicine. I have noticed lately that the other foot is starting. His toes turn under.

One morning he called me and said I'm falling. He got on his knees and had to crawl to get to the chair in the living room. It is also very hard for him to sit in the chair so I have to pull him up so he can get on his back and put his feet up on the sofa.

He is a very independent guy, but he never wants to go into a nursing home. I tell him I won't put him in one."

- Janet

"I made the mistake of taking my husband to assisted living. The promises were not kept. It is essential that physical therapy be constant. A weekend is enough to set them back several weeks. The swallowing is treated with thickened liquids and of course a speech therapist overseeing the meal time.

We have to use an extreme amount of patience and a lot of mind reading because he doesn't always express himself the way he is thinking. Sometimes he gets really angry but hasn't got violent, other than tear his shirts off because he can't get it off. His dreams and illusions are always about working or being able to get up and out of his wheelchair and go home. The next time he never wants to go home again."

- Geri Strehl

"When asked the question what she would suggest as advice for families with a Parkinson's disease member, my mom's suggestion was be very patient with them. This is because sometimes they are having difficulty saying something, it is okay in their head but their mouth won't cooperate, or they forget in the middle of a conversation.

My mom used to have a memory you would not believe, and was a very strong willed, independent woman that raised five children as a stay at home mom. She also had a husband that was a police officer who worked two other jobs just to support us. When she was 45 years old she went back to work as a 411 operator for General Telephone.

They are both retired, and have battled with different illnesses in their latter years. My mom became blind in her sixties due to maneculer bleeding and I believe she had Parkinson for at least 5-7 years before it was diagnosed correctly.

She started falling and had some personality changes. Since we were ignorant of Parkinson's disease we didn't recognize it, but knew something wasn't right with her. Being so independent it was hard to get her to listen to our concerns, plus HMO's don't encourage a lot of testing!

Because of this I would recommend to any families out there, the minute you see something that does not look normal for you parents usual behavior or abilities, even if they are older, get them tested immediately, so they can get on the medication as soon as possible.

This will save a lot of heartbreak for all concerned! Then stay connected no matter what!! Parkinson's disease truly affects behavior so don't let overreaction ruin your relationship with you family!!

My mom gets angry and frustrated a lot quicker than she used to, and cries faster than she would before. My sister suggested that we just have to give her time to regroup sometimes with encouragement and other times just leave her alone. Music seems to help a lot too! But most of all lots of LOVE!!!!!"

- Francine, Sylvia and MaMa Dee

"My sister was diagnosed with Parkinson's about six years ago - she was 55 years old. We are learning more and more about it all the time.

One thing we both feel is important is to know the symptoms of Parkinson's and check with a competent doctor. My sister hid her symptoms from all of us for several years. She thought her problems were due to getting older and gaining weight. She noticed a tremor in one hand, had problems getting up from a chair, and could hardly dress herself.

Now, with treatment, she dresses herself, goes up and down stairs easily, uses her treadmill regularly and generally feels much better.

When I asked her what she would give as advice, her first response was to accept the diagnosis and go from there. It has been hard for her to accept the fact that she has Parkinson's - particularly on good days.

As far as we know, there was only one family member who had Parkinson's and that was a great uncle. My sister was a person who hated to take pills and now she must take them (a lot of them) several times a day.

When she first started treatment, she became very depressed. Looking at Parkinson's as a non-killing disease has helped her. We know that there is no cure but we are hopeful.

There are times when she has a lot of involuntary movement, other days very little. We both feel the worst thing you can do is to not do anything. She knows that she won't die from Parkinson's and she lives each day knowing that there will be worse days coming.

In the meantime, she travels a little, visits her grandchildren, helps me with mine, and the two of us share the daily visits to our mother who is in a nursing home.   She still maintains her home, cooks every day, uses her computer, plays card games (mostly Yahtzee) with her husband, and puts jigsaw puzzles together.   We both feel that a positive attitude is necessary to live with Parkinson's.

In my opinion, the only mistake she made was in hiding the symptoms from her family and co-workers. Thank Goodness she did check with her doctor who referred her to a neurologist who recognized her disease immediately and began treatment. We are all so thankful that she is doing so well now."

- Barbara

"I would like to add one idea that has helped me communicate with my mother. My mother, Betty, was diagnosed with Parkinson's in the fall of 2005. We had no idea what was about to unfold in the months to come.

To make matters worse she was not taking the medication as ordered and by May fractured her hip and shoulder. That was actually a blessing as we had her in rehab and she made wonderful progress. My daughter-in-law was on staff at the rehab-nursing home facility.

To sum things up, she never returned home with my father George 86, and after 3 runs with UT infections, we are now seeing a more even plateau.

I attend a monthly care-givers group with my father and sister. During the December session, the leader/pastor of the retirement community read an insert from an article that has made each visit after that one session so much easier.

The article was about a mother and daughter trying to deal with the mother's Alzheimer's condition. They simply were not dealing with it and in denial of what was happening. When they stopped pretending and acknowledged the changes, it changed everything.

The very next visit was Christmas Day. Mom was very confused and excited at the same time about leaving her room and celebrating Christmas. For the first time, I said to my mother, "Mom you have Parkinson's and it is not safe for you to live with Dad at home. Dad lives on the farm and you live here at Swiss Village where it is much safer. I continued to fix my Mother's hair & make-up and she felt so much better about herself and we had a wonderful day.

This may sound so simple, but not only did it help our Christmas Day, it also helped both parent's accept and deal with the changes. It does seem to be getting easier, allowing yourself to grieve the loss of lifestyles is also a very necessary process."

- Linda from Indiana, USA

"My husband had a very difficult time accepting the fact that he has Parkinson's. It took a lot of patience, love, and caring to help him along. Most importantly, I learned that no matter what I did or said or tried to do to help him in every way, he still had to experience every stage of acceptance on his own.

We have all been there in some way in our lives where we just have to suck it up and get on with our lives. I would have to say that it took almost a year from the time of his diagnosis December 2005. But he did it and is very independent and happy.

The medication works as he only has tremors on the left side, his arm and leg. He is very mobile and does not need a walker or a wheelchair. So he does work full time, and does everything he's always done with the help of his friends and me. His friends pick him up and take him out weekly. I do all the driving for doctors' appointments, etc.

In the past year together we have learned that everything has to be planned. We have daily routines for everything, always knowing hour to hour what exactly is needed to get through the day smoothly. I always have to think ahead because he gets very anxious about everything no matter how big or small. I work full time also, so he can't rely on me solely, and he wants to be independent.

We recently learned that he has severe sleep apnea. The doctor feels that once he gets this under control it will help elevate his exhaustion."

- Anonymous

"Sometimes I feel like I could write a book about our journey through the mountains and valleys of Parkinson's. Since time is of the essence I will offer only a few thoughts.

The most important thing I can tell people is never forget that the person you are now taking care of is still that man/woman you fell in love with. Never let them doubt for a minute that you still think of them in that manner. Cherish them in all aspects. Make sure they know early on that during the times you become frustrated as a caregiver (and you will) that you aren't frustrated with them, but with the darned disease.

Remember to laugh together. Maintain a sense of humor about the situations you find yourselves in. If there is anything you had wanted to do as a couple, do it before it's too late; a cruise, a vacation of any type - do it even if you have to borrow the money. The memories are a wonderful balm to the loneliness.

My husband died at the age of 59. He had MSA/Parkinson's for 11 or so years and I was blessed to be his wife for 10 of those years.

A couple of tips before I close. I bought a battery operated doorbell and put the base unit in the central part of the house. I then velcroed the buzzer part to my husband's wheelchair. I also attached a piece of Velcro to the nightstand by his bed. That way we could attach the doorbell there when he was in bed. This had a pleasant chime sound and was very helpful in him letting me know he needed me.

When it got to the point he couldn't stay upright in his chair, we bolted a race car harness to the chair. This was quite beneficial in keeping him upright. Much better than the regular seat belt that came with the chair. It had a quick release latch on it and was easy for him to undo when he wanted to get in bed.

I bought a toddler's toy that had the letters of the alphabet on it and when you pushed one it would say that letter. When Bob became unable to speak very loudly at all, we used this for him to communicate with us.

Another tip is I bought inexpensive T-shirts in all colors, cut the arms off and then cut the shirt up the sides. When we would go out to eat I would take one of these that matched the predominate color of his shirt. We would slip it over his head and it wasn't that noticeable that he had a "bib" on."

- Sharron Hutchins from Lindale, Texas, USA

"When my father was found to have Parkinson's the doctor told us to prepare for him to be in a wheelchair and we did. The expensive ELE wheelchair we purchased only worked for about 6 months as he was unable to judge distance and work the toggle.

Medicare will not help to get him a regular chair as they already helped get the ELE one. So save the money and just get the regular chair.

Also the doctor did not prepare us for the loss of memory that came with Parkinson's. We are now looking at placing him in a home after we had their house built to accommodate the wheelchair and his care until his passing.

He is living in the past a lot and his short term memory is shot. It is creating many arguments as to where he lives, he wants to go home, and he still thinks he is working and he has been retired for 20 years. He is still looking for his car and truck to the extent of trying to call the police to report them stolen.

I love my father very much and am prepared to care for him until he passes. His attitude towards us has changed from the loving father, to the person who thinks we steal his belongings and lie to him about our selling them. It has gotten so bad we are now considering placing him in a home.

Good luck to all who have this unfair card dealt their way in life. We have contacted a Senior Care Advisor to get help with the finances and get the help we need to get him into a home. This has been our best call so far. They know all the hoops to jump to get the most out of Medi-Cal and the VA. God be with all who have to deal with this."

- Jacque White

"The way I have been helping my husband to deal with his PD is to keep him busy. There are days when he is stiff, sore and thoroughly down but thankfully these are few and far between.

He now takes care of all the meals at home, planning and preparing. It takes him time but gives him a great sense of achievement. He often has to sit at the stove when his legs are bad but he feels he's making a contribution and this in itself is valuable when he is no longer able to work.

Thankfully he is still able to drive so he goes off to town for the items he needs for dinner etc so each day he has something to plan and occupy him.

I own a horse and every weekend we go off - me on the horse and he on his bike and manage 5 miles or so. Very occasionally he only feels like going a short way so we meet back at the yard and I find that he has already started on the stable chores.

He has a stool in the stable and tack room so he is able to sit down when his legs feel weak. He is also in charge of meals for Callum (our horse) and keeps a note of what we are running low on. I am sure Callum is receiving rather larger meals than I would probably give him but again, my husband feels involved and useful.

He thoroughly enjoys visiting the yard and interacting with everyone there. They are aware of his PD and make every effort to encourage him and also watch him in case he needs a hand but make sure he isn't aware of it. In fact the last 18 months or so that he has been involved with Callum, they all think he looks stronger and is certainly walking better.

I think the exercise is keeping his legs strong and encourages him to keep going rather than sit in a chair and mope."

- Evaline

"It has been a rather unique experience to go from daughter to caregiver of my Dad. On the down side, it saddens me to see my Dad need help. On the up side, I have become reacquainted with my Dad, his personality, and his sense of humor.

I pray for breakthroughs that will eradicate this disease and its debilitating aspects. I thank God for my Dad's health to date. I believe he needed help before he admitted it to anyone, and possibly for quite some time prior to our becoming aware of the severity of the problem.

To date, we have been able to provide care for Dad in-home, but as his steps become more labored and he sometimes is unable to walk, we are seeking alternate methods of care. My sisters and I want the best and safest care available for him. Getting information on care options is sometimes time consuming and exasperating.

Best wishes to all those folks who may read this. May God bless your special person with Parkinson's and all the people who care for our loved ones!"

- Anonymous

"What I would like to share with others is my experiences as the daughter of someone who has Parkinson's - my mother. She is 57. My parents live in a rural community in West Texas, far, far away. There are no major cities in any direction that don't require 3 to 4 hours of driving. Their town doesn't even have an airport.

My brother and I live and work in Dallas, Texas. My mother sees a neurologist in Dallas that I researched carefully, and she sees him every quarter for follow ups. This requires that she buy a bus ticket to get to the nearest city which has an airport - Midland Texas. That's a 3 hour shuttle ride. Then she boards a flight from Midland to Dallas and I pick her up at the airport and she stays a couple of nights, goes to the appointment, and then heads back the same way.

My brother and I sometimes split the cost of the ticket, and we treat my mom like a queen when she's here visiting. The traveling used to be very hard on my mother, especially when she went through bouts of depression and delusions caused by some of her medications. When she wasn't well, my dad would have to make the drive across the state (9 hours) to bring her here because it's cheaper for them to drive than purchase plane tickets. I once had to go and bring her to Dallas myself when she was having a crisis.

I guess I'm sharing all this with you because it has been a real struggle for my family. It's been taxing, especially when my mother is delusional or depressed. No psychiatrist or neurologist has been able to explain if it's due to meds or an underlying mental disorder that can be mild to severe at times.

I tell people that finding a good neurologist is like shopping for shoes, you don't just settle for the first pair you see, you have to try them on and several others before you pick the one you want to buy. That's been the case for us. My mother was seen by neurologists that we felt weren't meeting her needs, and it finally took looking in the big city across the state to find one that finally worked and improved the quality of her life.

Don't give up on finding a good doctor and don't stay with one that you aren't completely happy with. My mother is doing better these days because she has a routine at home and feels needed and safe. I love my mother more than anyone and would do anything to make her happy and comfortable.

I hope my story will inspire other caregivers to have strength and to have hope, as well as compassion for the patient and the caregivers."

- Erika Castillo, RN, from Dallas, Texas, USA

"Since my wife was diagnosed with PD a year ago I have been reading as much literature as I can. Hopefully experiences and little tips will help others with PD. When my wife found out she had PD she immediately took on the challenge that she was not going to let it interfere with her quality of life. She has been a very healthy woman for all of her 70 years. She was an excellent tennis player and downhill skiier. After her rehab of two knee replacements two years ago she was met with the PD diagnosis.

In order to keep her quality of life she has turned to her prior active life in the world of physical fitness. This is her program in a typical week. Each day she is at the health club. She plays double tennis twice a week, Yoga 3 days a week, Pilates 1 day a week, and water aerobics 3 days a week.

Needless to say she is a very active person and plans to continue this schedule week after week.

Currently she is on the minimum dosage of Sinemet 3 times a day. She really can't tell whether it helps or not since she feels no difference. She feels good with the exception that she has a tremor in her left hand.

She may have had PD 3 years prior to the diagnosis before the physician confirmed it. She does not complain about stiffness, shows no sign of slowness or balance. The meds don't seem to have side effects or on or off symptoms.

We don't know what would happen if she stopped her exercise program, but we believe that "if you don't use it, you loose it". That's been her motto to keep her going. The neurologist has said she is in the group that PD progresses slowly, whatever that means.

I guess the only tip that I have to offer is to continue an aggressive exercise program and evaluate how it affects future PD symptoms.

She still does not believe she has PD. Hopefully not."

- Ron Geromini

STORIES ABOUT DBS

"In 1986 at aged 40, to my great shock and disbelief I was diagnosed with Parkinson's disease.

After a referral to a neurologist, I was put on medication (details of which escape me now as this has been changed many times through the years).
I continued to work until 2001 but at that stage I was finding it almost impossible to continue as the effectiveness of the medication was decreasing rapidly and my 'on' periods were very much reduced, even though I was taking about thirty tablets daily.

Two separate neurologists advised me to have DBS surgery, saying that I would be a very suitable candidate as it would alleviate the dyskinesia (which was extremely bad) and it would give me a better quality of life.

In July 2004, my neurologist referred me for assessment to a hospital specializing in neurosurgery. The outcome of the cognitive and memory test would determine my suitability for DBS. I passed this test and later that day and through the night I was taken off all medication which was very unpleasant and uncomfortable.

About lunch time the next day, following my movement assessment, I was put back on medication again and allowed go home

In October 2004 I was admitted to hospital for DBS. My head was fitted with a steel type cage on the evening prior to surgery which was slightly uncomfortable. After surgery I was a bit disorientated but I understand this is quite normal. Thankfully, it didn't last too long.

My medication was reduced by 60% which I thought was a bit drastic, but it was later increased.

About three days following surgery, the PD nurse programmed the stimulator but she had enormous difficulty getting a suitable setting for my right side and even with the chosen settings, I didn't feel any overall improvement apart from the demise of the dyskinesia.

With regard to the stimulator, things haven't improved very much since surgery. I have been in and out of hospital several times since - monitoring my medication, adjusting the stimulator etc., but nothing seems to work. If I didn't have the surgery maybe I would be a lot worse.

I have just returned from another grueling week in the hospital. They are now saying that the location of the stimulator may not be in the best place to receive the most benefit. They have suggested adjusting it which would involve further surgery.

I am considering this!!"

- Kate from Wex.

"I don't remember exactly how I came to be diagnosed, but when my doctor said he suspected Parkinson's, I really didn't know anything about it. So I guess I wasn't smart enough to be depressed.

That was in 1996, as I recall, and he referred me to a neurologist who confirmed the diagnosis, or at least the suspicion. The only method to rule out similar maladies was to prescribe Sinemet, and if it gave relief, we could assume it was Parkinson's. He informed me the only *sure* way to be certain was to examine my brain after death. I decided to try the first method, and we started with small doses of Sinemet, and an agonist called Eldapryl.

I really think he suspected Parkinson's when he noticed my handwriting was worse than his. That and a constant tremor were the only indications at the time. These progressed to "freezing", and involuntary movements of head and limbs. Sinemet and other meds were gradually increased, until I was taking a liquid mixture of ten Sinemets a day, dissolved in water.

I attended Support Group meetings and so many neurologists' lectures I probably could have delivered Dr. Rezak's talk this morning, but not as well.

By Nov. of '04, I was taking so much medicine I wasn't sure whether my shaking was the result of Parkinson's or dyskinesia from the Sinemet. And I frequently "froze"; that is, I had to have help getting started walking. Also, my head constantly bobbed, and my legs moved uncontrollably. I couldn't drive because I was constantly sleepy.

Somewhere about there, I decided to take the plunge. Some doctors recommend doing one side at a time, I'm sure for good reason, but I opted to get it over with. Patience may be a virtue, but it's not one of mine.

On Nov. 17, I entered Alexian Bros. hospital for Deep Brain Surgery. I'll spare you the gory details, except to say I'm glad I had both sides done at once, because, like Boot Camp, I'm glad I did it, but wouldn't want to do it again.

Fifteen months later, I still can't walk as well as I'd like, but most other symptoms are under control - when I remember to take my meds on schedule."

- Bob Maxey

"I was diagnosed with Parkinson's 15 yrs. ago and it has steadily progressed since then. I can no longer write but I thank God for computers or else I'd really find it hard. At first it was only my left side that was 'doing it's thing' and as it got worse my neurologist suggested that I might want to consider getting a DBS and he referred me to a neurosurgeon in Vancouver.

He said I was a candidate for the operation and he explained it all to me. I was terrified at the idea and when we returned home I spoke to several people who had spouses or friends go through it and they all discouraged me from getting it done. So when I was called to go to VGH (Vancouver General Hospital) for the surgery I told them that I had changed my mind after speaking with three different people about it.

That was in March 2002 but by August I could barely control my left leg and arm and it was strongly suggested that I reconsider having the DBS, so this time I agreed to it. Naturally, I was a nervous wreck and our friends all came over with pizza and other goodies to wish me well and they told me I was the "bravest" person they knew. Well I'm not too sure about that but I am sure that we have some very wonderful friends whom I couldn't live without.

Once I arrived at the hospital for some strange reason my anxieties began to lessen. I don't understand why that happened but I was grateful for it as I managed to get a good night's sleep.

They took me down for surgery at about 7 am and as the doctor froze my head in four different sites, he said, "This will sting." Well he wasn't whistling Dixie! He screwed the halo onto my head in four places and then I had to get an MRI done. I hate this at the best of times as I'm claustrophobic and going into that tube with a halo on sure didn't make things any easier.

What really cracks me up though is when they tell you not to take any of your drugs from the night before and then when you get the MRI they tell a Parkinson's patient to "be still"............now to my way of thinking that's sort of like telling the tide, don't come in.

From there I was taken into the OR and they put a sort of cage thing over my head that seemed to have bars on the front. I suggested to someone that if they had a long, black cape I could go out on Halloween as the man in the iron mask.

This cage thing was then screwed down so that I was immobile from the neck on up, only my facial features could move. The doctor then shaved a patch of hair and froze my scalp and cut it open and that's when the drilling started. It was all very surreal; I couldn't believe that I was sitting there while someone drilled a hole in my head.

They finally got through and that's when he went in with the probe and he asked me if I could see stars. Yes I could and I could also feel pins and needles in my hand. I told him my left hand was shaking and he said he was doing that.

The next thing I knew I felt my whole left side just calm down and for the first time in years I was able to touch my thumb and little finger together. He seemed to go through that procedure a couple of times and that was it, all done.
I was so darn tired by this time and when they wheeled me back to my room my husbands' smiling face was the first thing I saw and I showed him, "Look what I can do!" I couldn't believe it was all over and I went home the next day.

When I had to see the surgeon for my 7 week check up he asked me if I'd gained any weight and I told him that I'd been gaining weight at about a pound a week and I figured at this rate Dave, my husband, would be soon taking me for a roll and not a walk. He told me the reason for the weight gain was because I wasn't doing 24/7 aerobics anymore.

The doctor was very pleased with how successful the operation had been. He told me I was in a very small percentage of people who achieved the results that I had. That was just over four years ago and up until now my left side has been doing very well. Things are starting to come back to it again as in the tremors and following the surgery my right side seemed to go to hell in a hand basket. At least I got over four good years, so that was something.

My right side is the one that's doing it's thing now and in September I started getting acupuncture and it seems to be helping somewhat to prevent the spasms I get so often. I'm not sure if it's the acupuncture that's doing it but Dave has commented that I don't seem to be getting as many spasms as I usually do, so I shall continue with them as they sure can't hurt.

I can't speak for others but I find if I am not sitting in a comfortable chair it seems to exacerbate the PD symptoms. Our friends all know this and I am always allowed to select the chair I find most comfortable, as I said, we are lucky to have such a wonderful group of friends.

I no longer drive and I miss that as much as not being able to write. However I have recently acquired a scooter and now can get out and about on my own. It's such a feeling of freedom. My hubby has put a clear strobe light on the front and a red strobe light on the rear of the scooter so as to make me more noticeable when I'm out running the roads. It's just nice to get out in the fresh air to blow the stink off."

- Elizabeth Boudreau from Comox, British Columbia, Canada

"Gosh... Sometimes I think I could write a book on that experience alone, if I could carve out the time. I'll just hit the high points. I hope and pray my Mom's (her name is Pat) experiences are atypical of DBS patients. In fairness to that technology, Mom had some things happen that may have affected any potential for it to work right from the start.

She had her surgery in March of 2005 to remedy her bilateral essential tremors, which had taken her to the point she could barely get a glass of water to her mouth with anything still left to drink. She was embarrassed to eat out in public, and being an extremely social person, that was not acceptable to her.

She had done some reading about DBS and contacted the ET Foundation. She had read materials that, of course, sang high praises and told stories of people who had the DBS procedure and had regained their independence and self-confidence - all that.

Mom had already pretty much decided she wanted to try the surgery by the time she talked with any of the rest of the family (she's a widow). Other than the shaking, she was fine - healthy, energetic, sharp of mind, self-confident and able to take care of herself. That's all changed.

Immediately after the surgery, we were in awe that her previously uncontrollable shaking had ceased. She had some speech impairment, some motor function/coordination issues, and some bouts of unpredictable emotions (laughing hysterically or crying for no apparent reason), but we were reassured that those would go away with time and therapy - both physical and speech.

The doctor told us that this was a "process", and that her impulse generators would need "tuning" over several visits before the maximum effect could be noticed. She did seem to improve each of the first couple "tune-ups".

It was during one of these "tuning" visits that a nurse/aide, while following directions from the doctor, appeared to turn a dial the wrong way or something on the machine used to set the magnitude of the impulses from the generators. This caused Mom to immediately stiffen and scream in agony, almost as if electrocuted.

The doctor immediately grabbed the controls and restored her settings to wherever they were before. Mom settled down but was in pain for several hours following that event. By the next day she was feeling better, but sore from the muscle contractions.

While she didn't seem to get worse, she also didn't seem to get better in terms of her speech, coordination, etc. She lived alone, and was doing okay on her own although she chose not to drive anymore. She had a couple minor falls due to her lack of coordination and balance, but nothing serious.

Until.....New Year's Eve Day 2005, she fell backward in her driveway and hit her head. I happened to be there and heard her cry out just before she hit the pavement. She was conscious but convulsing and not responsive. We called 911 and by the time the paramedics showed, she was conscious but had a horrible headache (go figure!).

Anyway, there allegedly was no damage to the DBS system, although she developed hydrocephalus over the next few weeks. They installed a brain shunt to drain the fluid off, but it also required "tuning" on a regular basis, allegedly toward some set point at which she would only require an annual check and perhaps minor adjustment.

The shunt was piped to her stomach and came loose three times, requiring more surgeries. We were told that it was not unusual for shunts to come loose and for them to have to be repositioned a few times. Thank God, after the third time, it is still in place. But each time, before they would conclude that a dislocated shunt was the problem, she would be disoriented, fall down, be moody, or whatever. And each time, she would recover only partially from where she had been before. By this time, they diagnosed her with "Parkinson's Plus", and Alzheimer's.

We had to move her to an assisted living facility in February 2006 as she fell a couple more times after the first serious fall on New Year's Eve Day. She continued to fall and deteriorate in other ways, so we moved her to a group home in October 2006.

She has much closer monitoring there, but even so, she fell again around the Christmas holiday in 2006, cracking her head wide open, and requiring about 30 stitches. She has, since the DBS surgery, whacked her head really good about 4-5 times.

She has continued to deteriorate. This past week or so she has become, for all practical purposes, unintelligible a good part of the time. When she can talk, she says it is difficult to articulate her thoughts, although she says she knows what she wants to say.

Her memory is going fast, especially short term memory. She is also having difficulty swallowing. As if she didn't have enough going on already, she also has GERDS, so when she eats, her food often tries to tries to come back up before it goes down. In a word, she is a mess.

Here is the thing -- and the purpose of my plea is to have readers beware: Because of the timing of these other events, we don't know – likely will never know -- if her condition is a result of the DBS surgery, the "over-cramping" in the doctor's office, the first fall, a combination of the falls, a stroke, Alzheimer's, or ?

Since Mom's surgery, I personally have only met one other person that had DBS done a couple years ago. He could not talk either, but his wife said that when he could, he said he would never have done it if he had any idea what it would do to him beyond getting rid of the shakes. Mom has said the same thing many times. If we could only reverse time....

This is likely more than you expected or wanted to know. It is hard to determine where to start and stop when telling the story. But hopefully, there is enough here to convince someone that they need to SERIOUSLY research this procedure for themselves and talk to people who have actually had it done before going down this path. And to know what the risks are beyond the flowery "success" stories many would have you believe. And to SERIOUSLY weigh the risks for themselves."

- Kenny

POEMS

"Nuisance"

To James Parkinson:

I have a strange condition
Called Parkinson's Disease,
I don't know where I got it from
Don't ask that question please!

It never used to bother me
Or affect the way I thought,
But as the years have passed on by
In a circle, I am caught.

I found the truth at forty one,
It was quite hard to take,
But I was absolutely sure,
They had made a huge mistake.

In my cruel diagnosis
It just could not be true,
So I tried hard to ignore it
The best that I could do!

After many years of silence
I had to start and tell,
This was not just for the old folks
But hit the young as well!

In trying to grin and bear it
Have taken the right path,
Not lost sight of the importance
To smile or have a laugh.

Now things have become annoying,
Frustration plays a part,
Wish my life to be mine again
Sound body, mind and heart.

But twenty four small pills a day
Are working to improve,
The way I feel about these things
And also how I move.

My head is full of feelings
It's hard to understand,
Is this the way it was meant to be
Just how my life was planned?

Is there a role I have to play
To make people aware,
Of what we need to live our lives,
A knowledge I can share?

Or shall I just go bury my head
And hope there'll be a cure?
To face a much brighter future
I wish I could be sure!

- Lindsey Priest from Hornsea, England

"Laugh and the World Laughs with You!"

Things can only get better.
Look on the bright side of life,
There are plans you are not aware of
As to how to live your life.

I know this is the truth now
Don't ask me to explain,
Only keep it to yourself
If you live your life in pain.

If they ask you how you are feeling,
Say 'Great. I'm doing good!'
Well that's the talk of youngsters,
You'd be one if you could!

Getting older is no joke now,
In fact it's as cruel as hell,
There's one thing that's for certain
It's for those who are feeling well.

Survival of the fittest,
It must be you not me,
I wish we could change places,
Open your eyes so you can see.

That's all, it's off my chest now,
Tomorrow will be fine,
Reassess the situation,
Give myself some space and time.

AND IF YOU'VE STAYED THE JOURNEY
OF THIS RATHER DREARY TALE
JOIN ME IN FITS OF LAUGHTER
A TONIC THAT WILL NEVER FAIL!!

- Lindsey Priest from Hornsea, England

"Tremor"

It began long before
Unnoticed, sinister, deep decay
Dry rot in the loft
Not a problem to anyone.....until the roof falls in

The first signs........butterfly kiss
On the margins of consciousness
Trembling hand......... on the edge of sight
A bat's squeak warning......building slowly to a scream

Funny thing........ wobbly hand
Must check it out.............tomorrow
Sure it's nothing...........odd though
Doctor doesn't laugh.........anxiety twists inside

Brain tumor?.........need a scan.....do some tests
Parkinson's Disease
Is this me?.........I don't think so
Choking panic.........buried quickly beneath a cloak of normality

Future folded away
Like an old telescope, concertina'd shut
Focus on the present
Deal with today............tomorrow is too scary a place
Stage one............business as usual
No problem.........not as yet.......denial
Dawning recognition
Something's wrong.....the sparks of sympathy ignite

Do I look that bad?
A London cabbie waives the charge
"Don't worry love, you have a good day"
DO I LOOK THAT BAD? .....the icy blast of reality

Sympathy, so well meant, so resented
Yes I'm fine, no thank you, I'll manage
Furrowed concern......lighten up
Creeping dependency.........crave mindless fun

CAN'T DRIVE, CAN'T DANCE, CAN'T WALK FLUIDLY
CAN'T TASTE, CAN'T WRITE, CAN'T STAND THE CHANGE I SEE
CAN'T COMPLAIN OR CONFIDE OR I'LL BE THOUGHT A MISERY
CAN'T BEAR TO IMAGINE WHAT THE FUTURE HOLDS FOR ME

Ratcheted stiff and stooped
Tottering, unsteady and inept
Cramped muscles, restive ache
Wearisome effort....turning in bed.....cutting up food

Spiteful, mean, cruel disease
The road ahead is always steeper
The load gets ever heavier
And those you love must take another path

Resting leaden limbs, envy stabs deep
Effortless, unappreciated competence all around
Gone forever for me
Yet with its loss I see......I am, I have, I CAN

Compromise and adjust
Turn to swim with the flow, live for today
Dwell on the good and the bad recedes
It is me.....
...why not me....
.....believe me....
...won't beat me.

"A Time to Be Still"

Take my hand I know it's shaking
I know why your heart is breaking
Our love is strong and we'll get by
I know your sad but please don't cry
We'll fight this thing through thick and thin
I know my love, we'll not give in
Your help and love will see me through
You by my side I'll know just what to do
Hand in hand, we'll face each test
Day by day we'll make the best
A time to laugh, a time to cry
A time to stare it in the eye
Keep your faith, keep your will
A time to move, a time to be still

Parky's got me and he's cruel
He's really mean and needs no fuel
There's no respect for race or creed
He's got no habits, got no greed
He'll make you falter make you fall
Take your sleep can't smile at all
Hell make you stoop, he'll make you shake
He'll give you nothing, only take

We'll be a team, fight as we ought
Look out Parky your time is short
Doctors and Nurses will keep you at bay
Good people working for your judgment day
Hang on Parky's it won't be long
We'll have a party, sing a song
And when you're gone we'll have a ball
We'll say good riddance one and all
We'll be free.

- Bryn Davies

ARTICLES

"Could Your Bathroom Habits Increase Your Risk of Parkinson's?"

Date of Article: 03/03/2006

"Did you know that the number of times you visit a bathroom every day can determine your risk of Parkinson's disease? I know it sounds crazy, but it's true. I had a patient several years ago who suffered from an extreme case of Parkinson's disease. But, strangely enough, she would make a dramatic recovery any time she had a bowel movement. One day she could walk around and function quite normally. The next day, though, she would have advanced Parkinson's-like symptoms. Then she would completely recover a few days later.

This patient insisted that as long as she moved her bowels, she remained functional. If she missed a day, she would become rigid and have typical tremors of advanced disease. An enema would promptly clear it. The case was so clearly associated with constipation it made me wonder: Could Parkinson's and constipation possibly be related? And sure enough....

As part of an ongoing long-term (24 years) study, a research group recently confirmed what I've long suspected. They found that many cases of Parkinson's disease can be linked directly to constipation.

Over 8,000 men participated in the study. The researchers divided the men into four different groups according to how many bowel movements they had each day (less than one, one, two, more than two). Their results showed that your risk of developing Parkinson's is four-and-a-half times greater if you have less than one bowel movement per day versus having more than two.

The authors believe that degeneration in the central nervous system causes constipation. And as that degeneration progresses, it might also lead to Parkinson's.

I have a different theory: I think the constipation itself leads to damage to your nervous system. Here's why: I've long known that bacterial toxins absorbed into your bloodstream from your gut will directly attack the cells in your nervous system. We also know that pesticides contribute to the development of Parkinson's. This study reconfirms suspicions that toxins damage these controlling nerve cells.

Millions of men and women are developing this crippling disease. By the time symptoms manifest, the damage has been done. I believe the majority of cases can be prevented. All you have to do is eat organic foods, which eliminate your intake of pesticides, and increase the amount of fruits and vegetables in the diet.

This gives you better bowel function and larger stools, minimizing the amount of time the toxic material is in contact with your colon.

You can get additional protection by taking plenty of antioxidants, particularly vitamins C and E. I also recommend the mineral selenium. All of these help maintain and recycle abundant levels of glutathione, your body's principal detoxifier. And, finally, reduce your heavy metals and iron with chelation therapy.
The best management of Parkinson's disease, like most chronic degenerative conditions, is prevention. It doesn't have to happen!

Yours for better health and medical freedom."

- Robert Jay Rowen, MD

"Current research links MSG to neurodegenerative diseases like Alzheimer's, Huntington's, Parkinson's, and Amyotrophic Lateral Sclerosis (ALS).

FDA records show that MSG was never actually tested, but it was given an automatic GRAS (generally regarded as safe) status as were salt and pepper in the 1950s.

Children and elderly are most vulnerable to the degenerative effects of MSG. Here is a brief list of common effects of MSG and some curious statistics published by national organizations.

Heart maladies- More than 70 million Americans have one or more forms of cardiovascular disease and 43% of all deaths in the U.S. are related to these problems. The number of cardiovascular operations went up 287% from 1980-1990.

Alzheimer's disease, not an identifiable healthcare cost in 1980, now ranks third after cancer and heart disease among the most costly health problems in America. Four million people afflicted at a cost of $47,000/person/ year is $188 billion/year in healthcare costs.

Headaches & Migraines- $2.2 billion/year are spent on drugs to treat headaches, with a 74% increase in these chronic conditions between 1980 and 1990.

Asthma, which was on the decline until the mid-eighties, now shows a 100% increase in the death rate among children and seniors. Incidence has increased 600% in the last 10 years. The FDA recognizes that uncontrollable asthma" can be caused by MSG, but stops there, unfortunately.

Tumors – There has been an 88% increase in tumors since 1982. Birth Defects and Reproduction Disorders - MSG is a known mutagen (mutates fetuses) and causes significant damage to intellectual development, growth patterns, reproduction and gonadal functions.

Neurological/Emotional Disorders - Lab studies show devastating effects on brain development including dyslexia, autism, attention deficit disorder, hyperactivity, schizophrenia, violent episodes (rage), panic attacks, seizures, paranoia, depression, and cerebral palsy. Humans are 5 times more sensitive to MSG than rats which were used in tests.

Obesity is one of the most consistent effects of excitotoxin exposure and is a growing problem, nationwide, that knows no age or sex boundaries. In fact, scientists feed glutamate to young laboratory animals as a reliable way of inducing obesity. MSG triggers an insulin/adrenalin/fat storage/food craving response. This depletes serotonin levels which trigger headaches, depression, fatigue, and leads to more food cravings.

Fibromyalgia is a growing epidemic. Fibromyalgia patients who eliminated MSG and aspartame during a study conducted by the University of Florida reported complete relief of symptoms (2001).

Parkinson's, ALS, MS, and Huntington's diseases, like Alzheimer's, are all progressive neurogenic diseases showing brain/nerve cell damage.

Other symptoms of MSG sensitivity include: swollen throat and tongue, racing heart, joint pain, vertigo, skin disorders, sleeping disorders, burning, tightness or redness on face, and gastrointestinal complaints.

Tests and Misinformation Dr. Adrienne Samuels (Ph.D. in Research) in a 1999 industry journal ("Accountability in Research") stated that human tests of MSG, ... were often poorly designed, included inaccurate data and came to misleading conclusions." She wrote, "flawed research, suppression of facts and dissemination of inaccurate information are all tools that are used by special interest groups to mislead the public and government agencies."

Her research showed that all tests to date have been funded by or had ties to the food industry. These lobby groups are comprised of the largest food companies in America who profit from MSG use."

For more information:

Books:

Battling the MSG Myth by Debby Anglesey

Excitotoxins: The Taste that Kills by Dr. Russell Blaylock, Neurosurgeon

In Bad Taste: The MSG Symptom Complex by Dr. George Schwartz

Toxicologist Fibromyalgia Study: www.theannals.com, (The Annals of Pharmacotherapy, 1 June 2001, Vol. 35, pp 702-706.)

Websites:

www.msgmyth.com
www.msgtruth.org
www.truthinlabeling.org
www.nomsg.com

With special thanks to: Wayne Erickson MSG Information Center

Extracted from: What is MSG?

"I wondered if there could be an actual chemical causing the massive obesity epidemic, so did a friend of mine, John Erb. He was a research assistant at the University of Waterloo in Ontario, Canada, and spent years working for the government.

He made an amazing discovery while going through scientific journals for a book he was writing called "The Slow Poisoning of America". In hundreds of studies around the world, scientists were creating obese mice and rats to use in diet or diabetes test studies. No strain of rat or mice is naturally obese, so the scientists have to create them. They make these morbidly obese creatures by injecting them with MSG when they are first born. The MSG triples the amount of insulin the pancreas creates; causing rats (and humans?) to become obese. They even have a title for the fat rodents they create: "MSG-Treated Rats".

I was shocked too. I went to my kitchen, checking the cupboards and the fridge. MSG was in everything! The Campbell's soups, the Hostess Doritos, the Lays flavored potato chips, Betty Crocker Hamburger Helper, Heinz canned gravy, Swanson frozen prepared meals, Kraft salad dressings, especially the 'healthy low fat' ones.

The items that didn't have MSG marked on the product label had something called "Hydrolyzed Vegetable Protein", which is just another name for Monosodium Glutamate. It was shocking to see just how many of the foods we feed our children everyday are filled with this stuff.

They hide MSG under many different names in order to fool those who carefully read the ingredient list, so they don't catch on. (Other names for MSG: 'Accent' - 'Aginomoto' - 'Natural Meet Tenderizer' etc.) But it didn't stop there.

When our family went out to eat, we started asking at the restaurants what menu items had MSG. Employees, even the managers, swore they didn't use MSG. But when we asked for the ingredient list which they provided, sure enough MSG and Hydrolyzed Vegetable Protein were everywhere.

Burger King, McDonald's, Wendy's, Taco Bell, every restaurant, even the sit down ones like TGIF, Chili's, Applebee's and Denny's use MSG in abundance. Kentucky Fried Chicken seemed to be the WORST offender: MSG was in every chicken dish, salad dressing and gravy. No wonder I loved to eat that coating on the skin, their secret spice was MSG!

So why is MSG in so many of the foods we eat? Is it a preservative or a vitamin? Not according to my friend John. In the book he wrote, an expose of the food additive industry called "The Slow Poisoning of America" he said that MSG is added to food for the addictive effect it has on the human body.

Even the propaganda website sponsored by the food manufacturers lobby group supporting MSG explains that the reason they add it to food is to make people eat more. A study of the elderly showed that people eat more of the foods to which it is added.

The Glutamate Association lobby group says eating more benefits the elderly, but what does it do to the rest of us? 'Betcha can't eat just one', takes on a whole new meaning where MSG is concerned! And we wonder why the nation is overweight? The MSG manufacturers themselves admit that it addicts people to their products. It makes people choose their product over others, and makes people eat more of it than they would if MSG wasn't added.

Not only is MSG scientifically proven to cause obesity, it is an addictive substance! Since its introduction into the American food supply fifty years ago, MSG has been added in larger and larger doses to the pre-packaged meals, soups, snacks and fast foods we are tempted to eat everyday. The FDA has set no limits on how much of it can be added to food. They claim it's safe to eat in any amount.

How can they claim it safe when there are hundreds of scientific studies with titles like these?:

'The monosodium glutamate (MSG) obese rat as a model for the study of exercise in obesity'. Gobatto CA, Mello MA, Souza CT, Ribeiro A.Res Commun Mol Pathol Pharmacol. 2002.

'Adrenalectomy abolishes the food-induced hypothalamic serotonin release in both normal and monosodium glutamate-obese rats'. Guimaraes RB, Telles MM, Coelho VB, Mori C, Nascimento CM, Ribeiro Brain Res Bull. 2002 Aug.

'Obesity induced by neonatal monosodium glutamate treatment in spontaneously hypertensive rats: an animal model of multiple risk factors'. Iwase M, Yamamoto

M, Iino K, Ichikawa K, Shinohara N, Yoshinari Fujishima Hypertens Res. 1998 Mar.

'Hypothalamic lesion induced by injection of monosodium glutamate in suckling period and subsequent development of obesity'. Tanaka K, Shimada M, Nakao K, Kusunoki Exp Neurol. 1978 Oct.

Yes, that last study was not a typo, it WAS written in 1978. Both the "medical research community" and "food manufacturers" have known about MSG's side effects for decades! Many more studies mentioned in John Erb's book link MSG to Diabetes, Migraines and headaches, Autism, ADHD and even Alzheimer's. But what can we do to stop the food manufactures from dumping fattening and addictive MSG into our food supply and causing the obesity epidemic we now see?

Even as you read this, G. W. Bush and his corporate supporters are pushing a Bill through Congress called the "Personal Responsibility in Food Consumption Act" also known as the "Cheeseburger Bill", this sweeping law bans anyone from suing food manufacturers, sellers and distributors. Even if it comes out that they purposely added an addictive chemical to their foods.
The Bill has already been rushed through the House of Representatives, and is due for the same rubber stamp at Senate level. It is important that Bush and his corporate supporters get it through before the media lets everyone know about 'MSG, the intentional Nicotine for food'.

Several months ago, John Erb took his book and his concerns to one of the highest government health officials in Canada. While sitting in the Government office, the official told him "Sure I know how bad MSG is, I wouldn't touch the stuff!" But this top level government official refused to tell the public what he knew.

The big media doesn't want to tell the public either, fearing legal issues with their advertisers. It seems that the fallout on fast food industry may hurt their profit margin. The food producers and restaurants have been addicting us to their products for years, and now we are paying the price for it.

Our children should not be cursed with obesity caused by an addictive food additive. But what can I do about it? I'm just one voice! What can I do to stop the poisoning of our children, while our governments are insuring financial protection for the industry that is poisoning us!

This email is going out to everyone I know in an attempt to tell you the truth that the corporate owned politicians and media won't tell you. The best way you can help to save yourself and your children from this drug-induced epidemic, is to forward this email to everyone. With any luck, it will circle the globe before politicians can pass the legislation protecting those who are poisoning us. The food industry learned a lot from the tobacco industry. Imagine if big tobacco had

a bill like this in place before someone blew the whistle on Nicotine?
If you are one of the few who can still believe that MSG is good for us, and you won't believe what John Erb has to say, see for yourself. Go to the National Library of Medicine, at http://www.pubmed.com Type in the words "MSG Obese" and read a few of the 115 medical studies that appear.

We the public, do not want to be rats in one giant experiment and we do not approve of food that makes us into a nation of obese, lethargic, addicted sheep, feeding the food industry's bottom line, while waiting for the heart transplant, diabetic induced amputation, blindness or other obesity induced, life threatening disorders.

With your help we can put an end to this poison. Do your part in sending this message out by word of mouth, email or by distribution of this article to all your friends all over the world and stop this 'Slow Poisoning of Mankind' by the packaged food industry.

Blowing the whistle on MSG is our responsibility, get the word out."

Extracted from: MSG Obesity & Health Alert